# HOLISTIC LIFESTYLE

THE APOTHECARY FARMACY SHOP

HEALTH & WELLNESS

CONSCIOUS EATING

SPIRITUAL WELLNESS

# BeUnique

MAGAZINE & RADIO

# CONTENTS

## CONSCIOUS EATING



## WELLNESS



## HOLISTIC SCIENCE NEWS



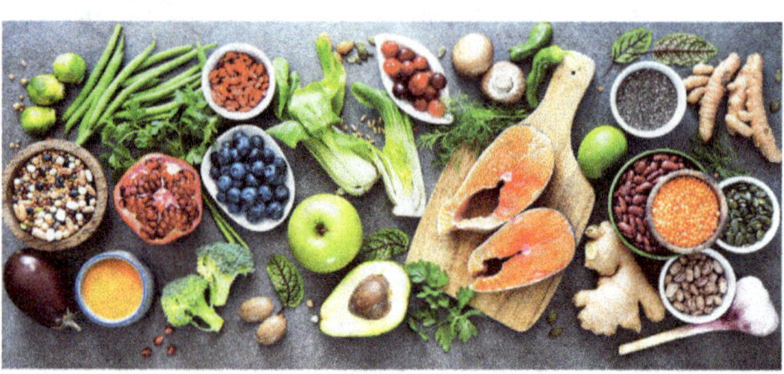

## SPOTLIGHT

*7 DAY PLANT-BASED MENU*

Great resource to help you plan your menu

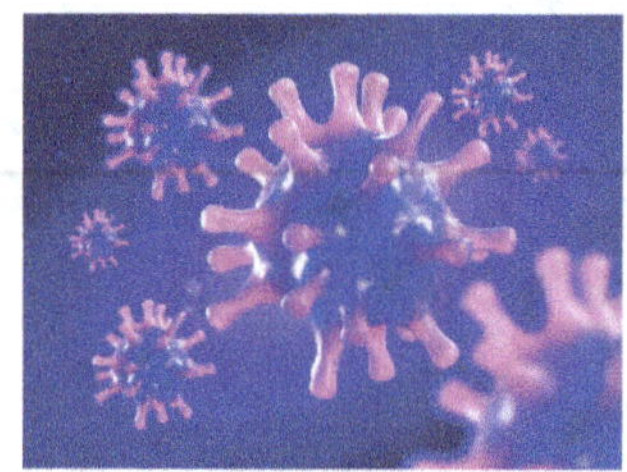

## WELLNESS

*SEAWEED EXTRACT OUTPERFORMS REMDESIVIR IN BLOCKING COVID-19*

New Science / p36

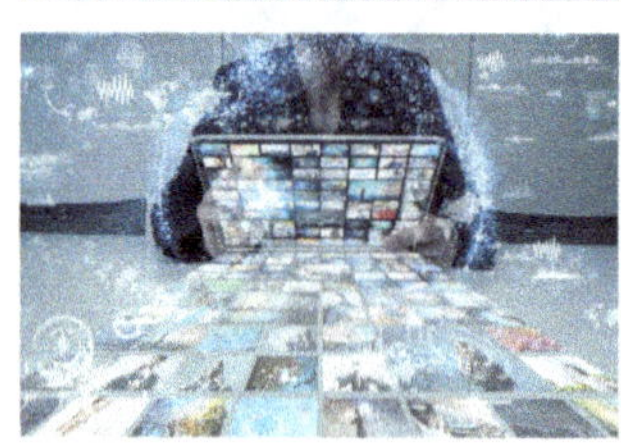

## MEDIA MARKETPLACE

*HOLISTIC MEDIA*

Check our new books ect / p50

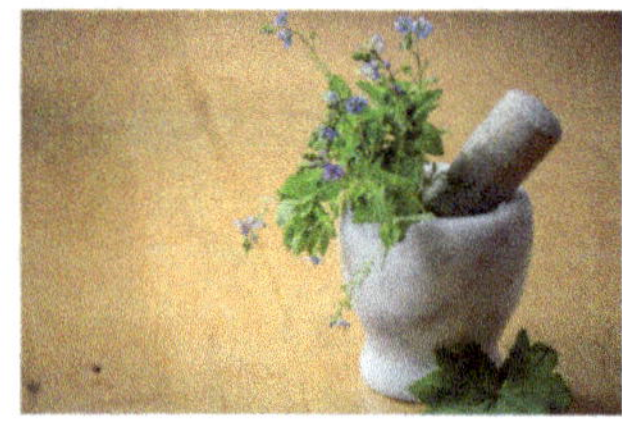

## HERBAL TIPS

*HERBAL LIFE*

A day in the life of Stella Young, and how she stays creative / p59

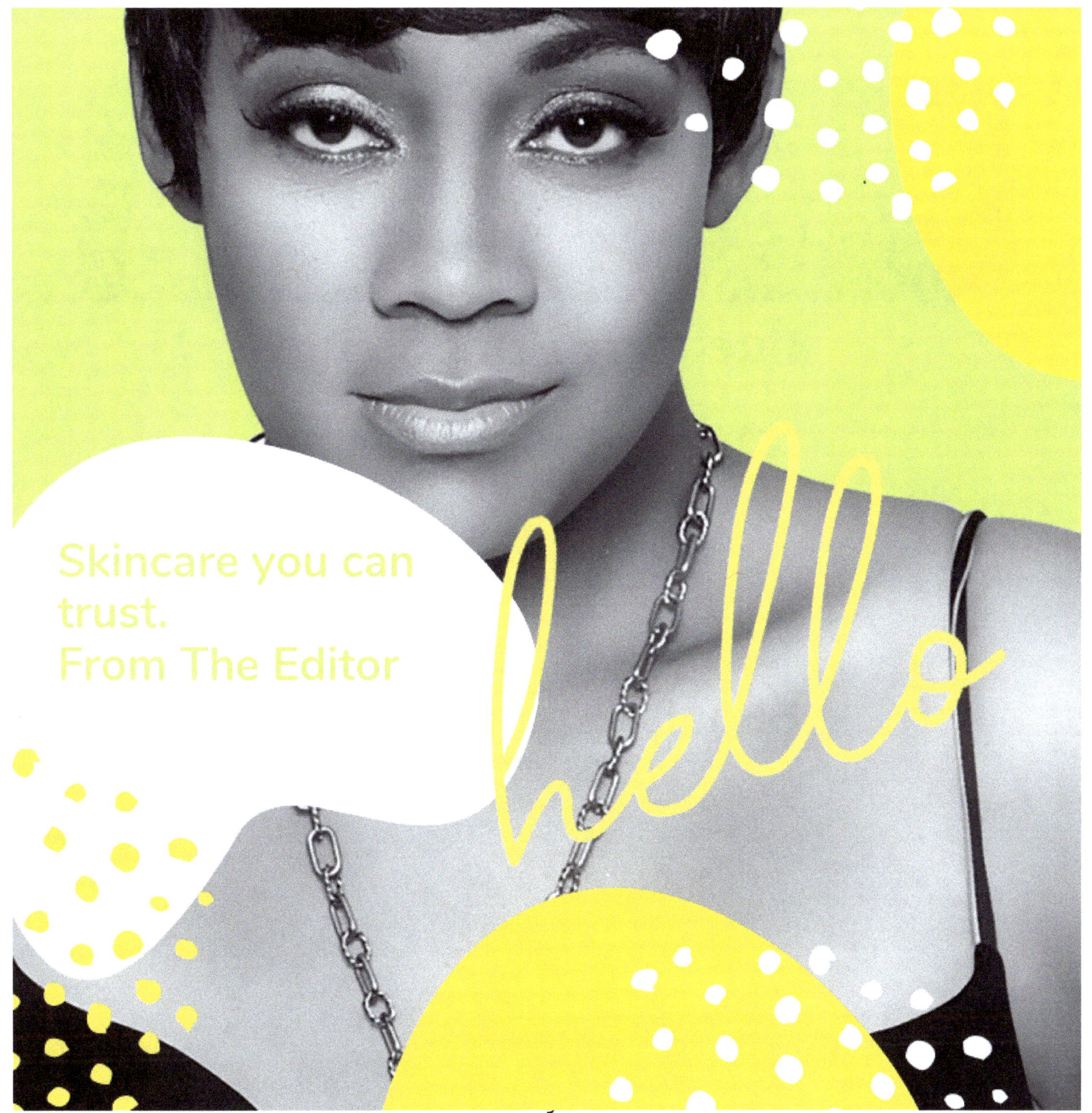
Skincare you can
trust.
From The Editor
hello

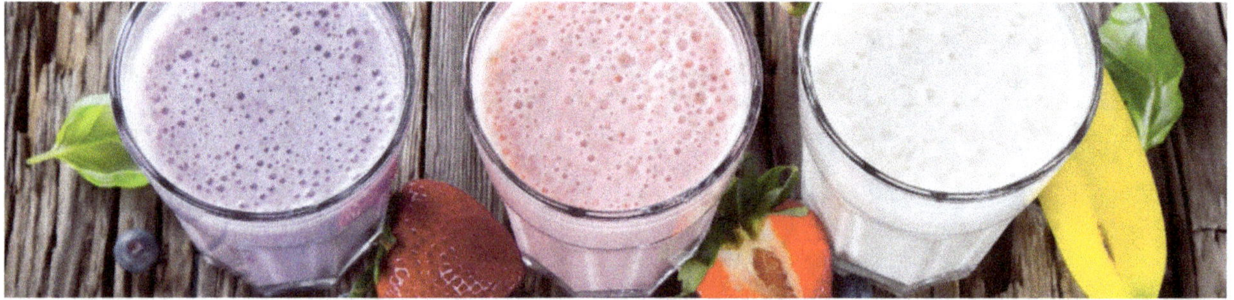

# Blueberry Fruit Shake

*2 Servings / 20 Minutes*

**Ingredients**

1 1/2 cups apple juice can substitute white grape juice, dairy milk, or almond milk
1 banana halved
1 1/2 cups frozen blueberries
3/4 cup vanilla Greek yogurt
fresh blueberries and mint sprigs for garnish optional

**Nutrition Facts**

Calories: 269kcal
Carbohydrates: 61g
Protein: 8g
Cholesterol: 2mg
Sodium: 34mg
Potassium: 561mg
Fiber: 4g
Sugar: 46g
Vitamin A: 100IU
Vitamin C: 17.6mg
Calcium: 22mg
Iron: 0.7mg

**Instructions**

♦ Place the apple juice, banana, blueberries and Greek yogurt in a blender.

♦ Blend until completely smooth.

♦ Pour into glasses and serve, topped with blueberries and mint if desired.

# Banana Fruit Shakes

*2 Servings / 40 Minutes*

**Ingredients**

1 1/2 cups pineapple juice
2 banana cut in half
1/2 cups frozen pineapple chunks
3/4 cup vanilla Greek yogurt
fresh pineapple wedges and mint sprigs for garnish optional

**Nutrition Facts**

Calories: 169kcal
Carbohydrates: 33g
Protein: 6g
Cholesterol: 2mg
Sodium: 33mg
Potassium: 744mg
Fiber: 7g
Sugar: 35g
Vitamin A: 250IU
Vitamin C: 62.7mg
Calcium: 91mg
Iron: 1.9mg

**Instructions**

♦ Place the pineapple juice, banana, frozen pineapple and vanilla Greek yogurt in a blender.

♦ Blend until smooth.

♦ Pour into 2 glasses. Garnish with pineapple wedges and mint sprigs if desired.

# Strawberry Banana Fruit Shakes

*2 Servings / 40 Minutes*

**Ingredients**

1 1/2 cups apple juice
1 1/2 bananas
1 1/2 cups frozen strawberries
3/4 cup vanilla Greek yogurt
fresh fruit and mint sprigs for garnish optional

**Nutrition Facts**

Calories: 206kcal
Carbohydrates: 60g
Protein: 8g
Cholesterol: 2mg
Sodium: 34mg
Potassium: 746mg
Fiber: 4g
Sugar: 44g
Vitamin A: 55IU
Vitamin C: 72.8mg
Calcium: 32mg
Iron: 0.9mg

**Instructions**

- Place the apple juice, bananas, frozen strawberries and vanilla Greek yogurt in a blender.
- Blend until completely smooth.
- Pour into 2 glasses and serve, garnished with fruit and mint sprigs if desired.

---

# Mango Fruit Shakes

*2 Servings / 20 Minutes*

**Ingredients**

1 1/2 cups mango nectar can substitute a different type of juice such as apple or orange juice
1 banana cut in half
3/4 cup vanilla Greek yogurt
1 1/2 cups frozen mango chunks
lime slices and mint springs for garnish optional

**Nutrition Facts**

Calories: 188kcal
Carbohydrates: 47g
Protein: 8g
Cholesterol: 2mg
Sodium: 36mg
Potassium: 540mg
Fiber: 4g
Sugar: 37g
Vitamin A: 2680IU
Vitamin C: 78.8mg
Calcium: 46mg
Iron: 1mg

**Instructions**

- Place the mango nectar, banana, Greek yogurt and mango chunks in the blender.
- Blend until completely smooth.
- Pour until 2 glasses and serve, garnished with lime and mint if desired.

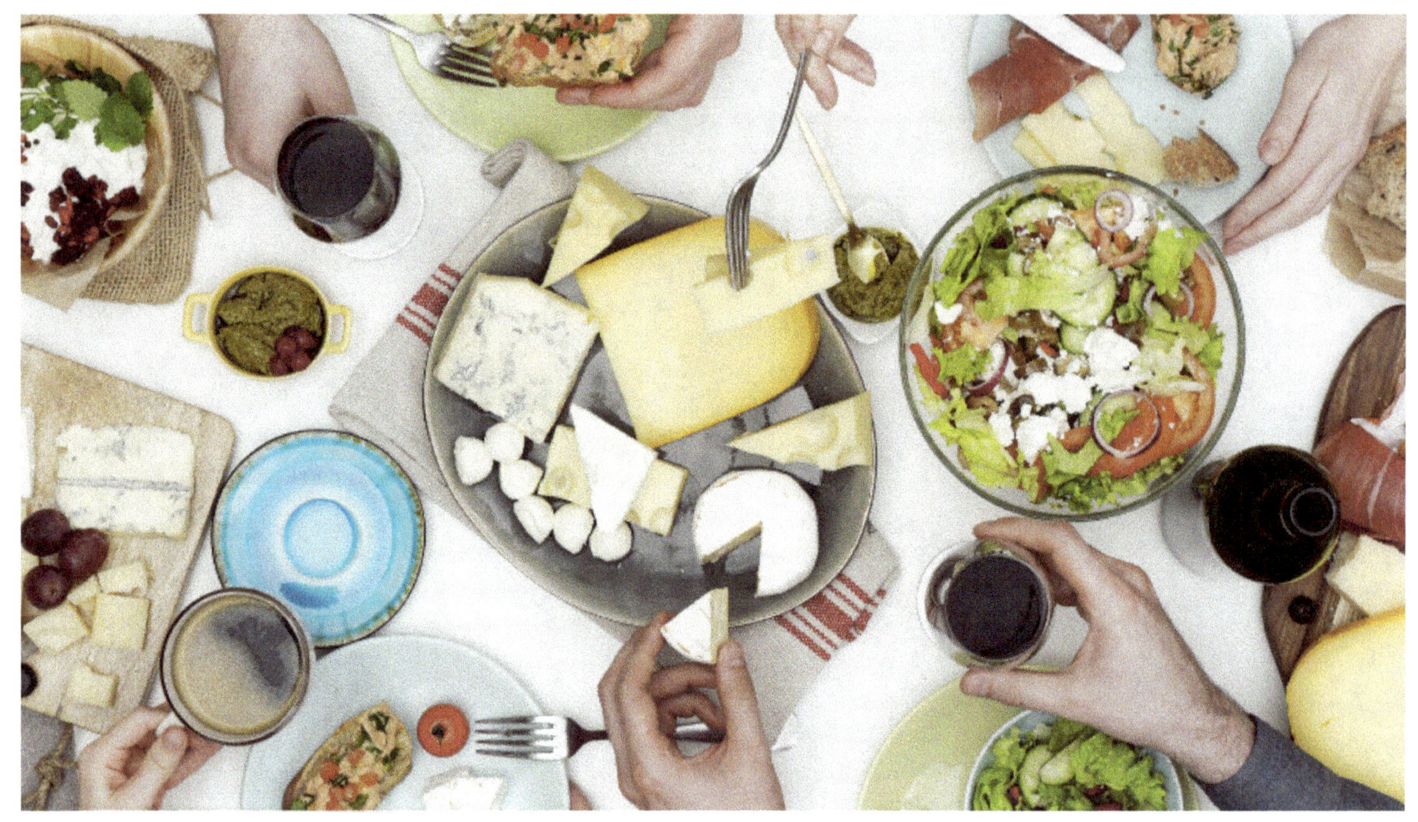

# 7 Steps to Conscious Eating

*According to a 2011 report from the U.S. Department of Agriculture, the average American spends two-and-a-half hours a day eating, but more than half the time, we're doing something else, too. Because we're working, driving, reading, watching television, or fiddling with an electronic device, we're not fully aware of what we're eating. And this mindless eating—a lack of awareness of the food we're consuming—may be contributing to the national obesity epidemic and other health issues, says Dr. Lilian Cheung, a nutritionist and lecturer at Harvard T.H. Chan School of Public Health.*

## What is Conscious eating?

Conscious eating includes Mindful eating is maintaining an in-the-moment awareness of the food and drink you put into your body, observing rather than judging how the food makes you feel and the signals your body sends about taste, satisfaction, and fullness.

*" The tenets of mindfulness apply to mindful eating as well, but the concept of mindful eating goes beyond the individual. It also encompasses how what you eat affects the world. We eat for total health,"*

DR. CHEUNG

## Mindful Eating

Mindfulness means focusing on the present moment, while calmly acknowledging and accepting your feelings, thoughts, and bodily sensations." The tenets of mindfulness apply to mindful eating as well, but the concept of mindful eating goes beyond the individual. It also encompasses how what you eat affects the world. We eat for total health," Dr. Cheung says. That's essentially the same concept that drove the development of the 2015 pro-posed U.S. Dietary Guidelines, which, for the first time, considered sustainability of food crops as well as the health benefits of the foods.

Although the ideal mindful-eating food choices are similar to the Mediterranean diet—centered on fruits, vegetables, whole grains, seeds, nuts, and vegetable oils—the technique can be applied to a cheeseburger and fries. By truly paying attention to the food you eat, you may indulge in these types of foods less often. In essence, mindful eating means being fully attentive to your food—as you buy, prepare, serve, and consume it. However, adopting the practice may take more than a few adjustments in the way you approach meals and snacks. In the book Savor: Mindful Eating, see the , Dr. Cheung and her co-author, Buddhist spiritual leader Thich Nhat Hanh, suggest several practices that can help you get there, including those listed below.

**1. Begin with your shopping list.**
Consider the health value of every item you add to your list and stick to it to avoid impulse buying when you're shopping. Fill most of your cart in the produce section and avoid the center aisles—which are heavy with processed foods—and the chips and candy at the check-out counter.

**2. Start with a small portion.**
It may be helpful to limit the size of your plate to nine inches or less.

**3. Appreciate your food.**
Pause for a minute or two before you begin eating to contemplate everything and everyone it took to bring the meal to your table. Silently express your gratitude for the opportunity to enjoy delicious food and the companions you're enjoying it with.

**4. Bring all your senses to the meal.**
When you're cooking, serving, and eating your food, be attentive to color, texture, aroma, and even the sounds different foods make as you prepare them. As you chew your food, try identifying all the ingredients, especially seasonings.

**5. Take small bites.**
It's easier to taste food completely when your mouth isn't full. Put down your utensil between bites.

**6. Chew thoroughly.**
Chew well until you can taste the essence of the food. (You may have to chew each mouthful 20 to 40 times, depending on the food.) You may be surprised at all the flavors that are released.

**7. Eat slowly.**
If you follow the advice above, you won't bolt your food down. Devote at least five minutes to mindful eating before you chat with your tablemates.

Welcome to Conscious Eating. What follows will not be a new dietary ideology, super food, or miracle cleanse. Rather, we will explore a life long, lifestyle approach to food based on the Ayurvedic Paradigm of Health.

Before we dive into the main course, however, here's a few observations on food and health throughout the ages. Even if you are unfamiliar with the quotes, you may recognize some the names:

*"Let food be thy medicine and medicine be thy food."*
Hippocrates

*"The first wealth is health."*
Ralph Waldo Emerson

*Each patient carries his own doctor inside him."*
Norman Cousins

*"No disease that can be treated by diet should be treated with any other means."*
Maimonides

**"There is no magic bullet. You gotta eat healthy and live healthy to be healthy. End of story."**

MORGAN SPURLOCK

*"There is no magic bullet. You gotta eat healthy and live healthy to be healthy. End of story."*
Morgan Spurlock

*"Eating comfort food isn't a reward — it's a punishment."*
Drew Carey

The Principle of Conscious Eating is about far more than WHAT we eat. Ultimately, our goal is to choose foods that support and sustain life, longevity and good health. In addition, what we eat should prevent us from experiencing illnesses and alleviate their symptoms, should they occur. Are your current habits around food, which include not only WHAT, but WHEN and HOW you eat, working well for you. Can you say, without hesitation, that the your food habits are leading to abundant physical mental and emotional health?"

The word Conscious comes from the Latin word, scīre, meaning, "to know" or "to understand," Conscious eating requires observation and attentiveness. We take on the role of observers or Ayurvedic detectives. This means paying attention to what, how and when you eat as well as your digestive experience.

According to Ayurveda, it's not a question of whether any particular food is 'good' or 'bad'. Rather, you learn to observe how YOUR body process what you eat. The answer falls, roughly, into two categories, positive and negative digestive experiences. During and after a positive digestive experience, you feel satisfied, grateful and full of energy. The negative kind leads to what is

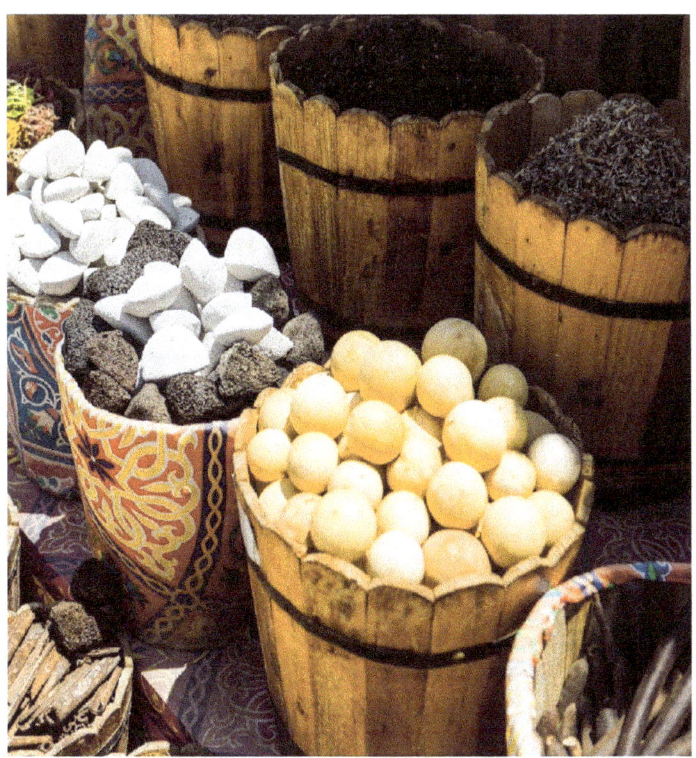

technically referred to as 'unhappy tummy'. Here, you may experience any or all of the following: bloating, gas, burning feeling, belching, lethargy and sleepiness.
Pretty big difference, huh?

Ayurveda sees the digestive tract as the "Master system" of the body. Food builds the physical body, mind and emotions. Just as every person is unique, all foods are not the same. Thus, generic diets, food plans, or cleanses WILL NEVER work for everyone. At best, these can only be effective for SOME of the people SOME of the time. This brings us to a simple truth, the definition of Conscious Eating: Continually Creating and Refining a Sustainable Eating Plan that Works for YOU.
This is a rich and, at times, complex practice. However, I will attempt to provide some basic Ayurvedic Principles and Guidelines in this article and the series of articles to follow. Are you ready?

THE BIG PICTURE ( The holistic Picture)
Conscious Eating, ultimately, is about our relationship with ourselves, our diet, and our environment. This includes: where we get our food, how it's grown, the manner in which it is prepared, the amount and timing of our meals, the people with whom we eat as well as our own behavioral and emotional patterns, that is, our beliefs and feelings about ourselves and whatever we eat.

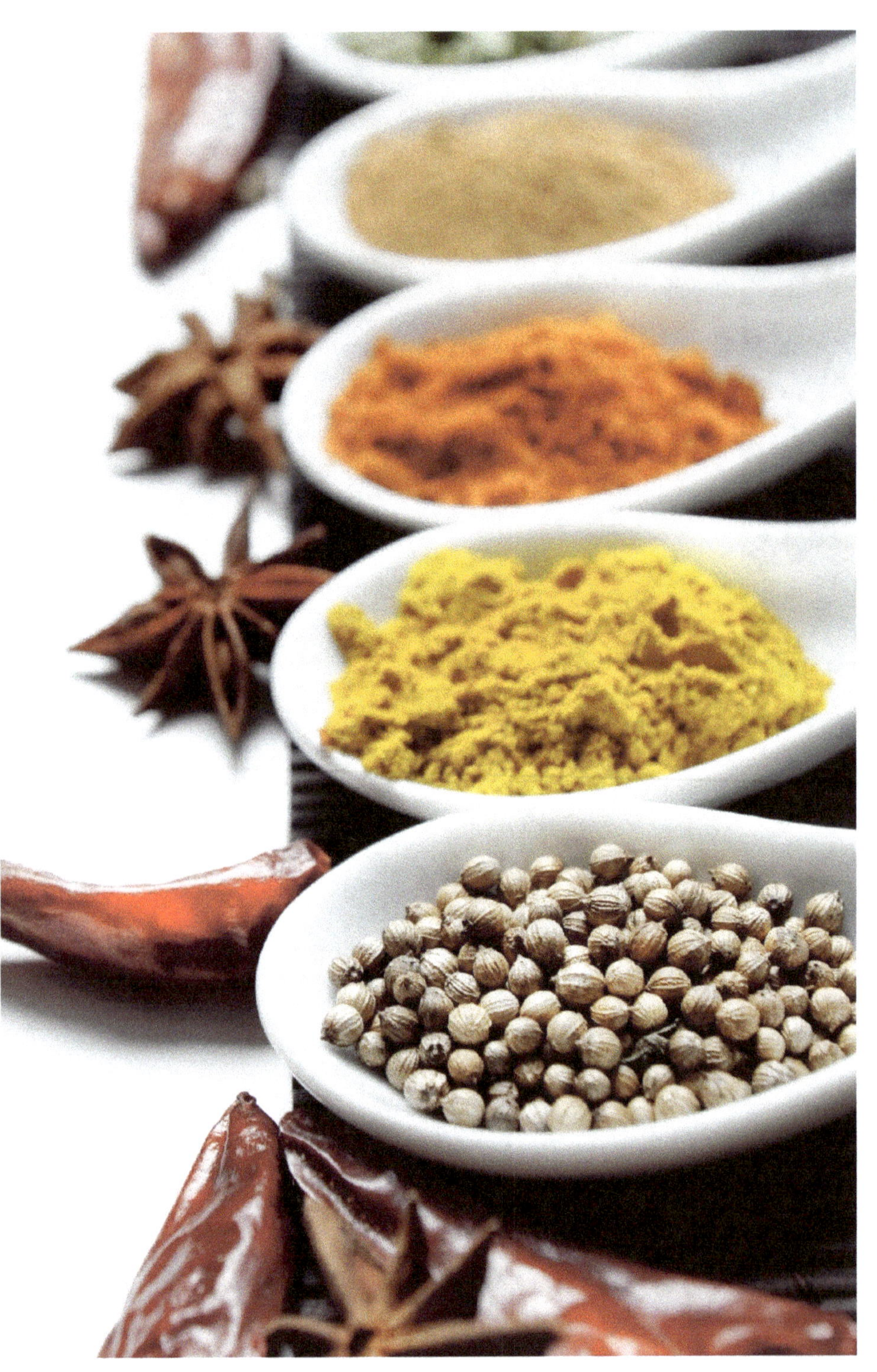

# Wealth is Health

## 6 Principles to Eating Consciously

To eat consciously, we need to work from the inside out. We begin by going beneath our habitual relationship with food and getting to know the energetics of food and digestion.

It is our own digestive experience that determines whether what we eat is supporting our body's metabolic processes or disrupting them. We have both the power and responsibility to create wellness and vitality. First, we must learn to read the subtle signs our body sends us. This includes our emotional states, as our diet directly affects our mood.

Conscious eating is when the individuals intake of food is supportive to health, vitality and wellbeing. My goal is that this becomes a lifestyle, a sustainable way of eating and living. Its our day to day habits over a long period of time that becomes our normal. If our habits are conscious, and moderate most of the time, then we steer ourselves on the path of health, because we take responsibility for our actions. With personal responsibility comes empowerment, which in turn leads to better understanding and choices. Its an upward spiral.

# 6 PRINCIPLES

**1. Your health is your most valuable currency**
Your body mind is your most valuable asset. If your are healthy and happy, then you can pursue your life's purpose. However, if you are tired, low energy or frequently sick, then most of your time is focused on thinking, identifying with and the treatment of your particular malady. Your good health is your most valuable currency, everything starts with you!!!! Seems to me that investing in my health is the highest priority. Physical health is dependent on what you eat. Start by investing your time and attention on the foods that make your body come alive with vibrancy. Conscious eating is one of the three pillars that support health, the other two being sleep and energy.

**2. Your Body/mind has to digest everything that comes in**
Every day you consume food and drink in response to hunger and other external cues with little thought to how, your body converts it. When your metabolic process is working efficiently, your body should utilize 70-80% of all food eaten. However, when digestion is insufficient, the body is not able to break down or use the food properly. Faulty digestion is the beginnings of your body's dis-ease.

Conscious eating is designed to educate and help you make connections with your digestive process.

**3. Take responsibility for your consumption of food.**
This means the types and amounts of food consumed and the timing of meals. Im sure you have noticed from observing your family and friends that we all have different relationships and need of food. How much or little we eat, the frequency of meals, the types of foods etc. An important key too good health is to eat the appropriate amount and types of foods that maintain great health for you. Your body uses everything you put into it. Over time symptoms such as fatigue, lethargy and sluggishness become the norm and the immune system suffers.

**4. The Burp is a practical exercise to rediscover your individual digestive capacity.**
Ayurvedic medicine states, that we should eat until we are not hungry. This is very different to eating until you are full.

"The stomach should be 1/2 filled by solid foods,
1/4 by water and 1/4 should be kept free for the movement of air"

The stomach naturally gives a burp when its three quarters 3/4 full.

Many of us have trained our stomachs to stretch by overeating or eating too frequently and this natural capacity has been overridden.

**5. Eat real food**
My greatest contribution to my health is that I love to prepare and cook my food.

I enjoy going to the farmers markets, searching for recipes and creating great food made with love.....nothing better. Hippocrates, the father of modern medicine said

'the forces within us are the true healers and food is the true medicine'

Eat a varied diet and buy the highest quality food you can. Mix it up and try a few vegetarian meals every week. Minimize meat and fish consumption. Try not to eat anything that comes in a box. Avoid or reduce all processed food, white sugar and trans fats. Instead create a diet based on plants, whole grains, beans, nuts, seeds and fruits. Get to know the foods that grow in your area and whats in season. When you eat seasonal, fresh, locally grown food, you deepen your connection with nature and your environment. As a result your body becomes revitalized.

**6. Use spices to enhance digestive and metabolic capacity**
Ayurveda recognizes that the foundation of good health rests on a healthy functioning digestive tract. Herbs and spices are used to enhance and support correct functioning of digestion and metabolism. Here we are using spices as medicine to correct, improve and regulate digestive fire. Spices can be used either before a meal to ignite the fire and increase digestion or after to facilitate the processing or metabolism of food.

In the next article I will discuss the burp and the three types of metabolic processes.

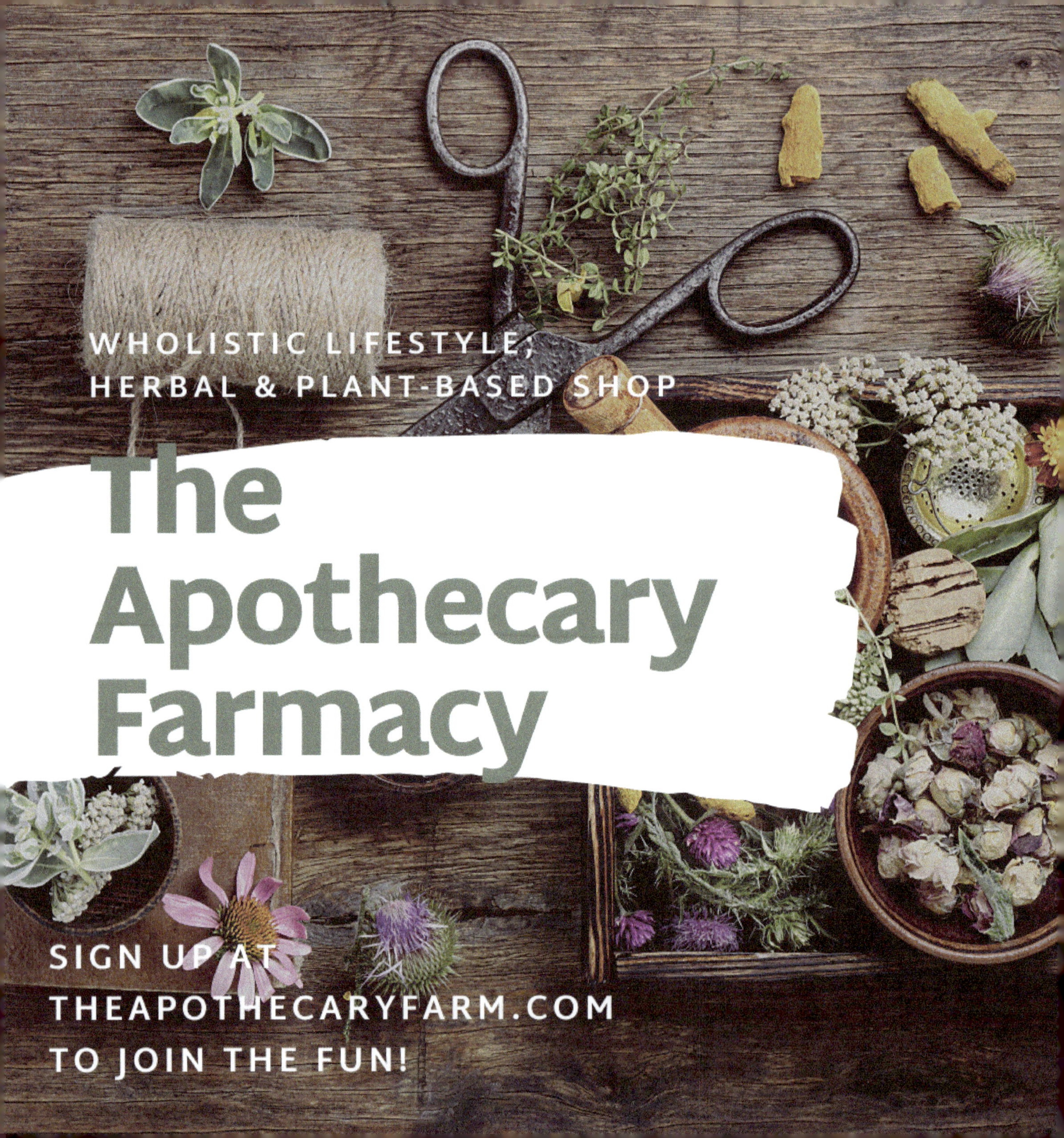
WHOLISTIC LIFESTYLE,
HERBAL & PLANT-BASED SHOP
The Apothecary Farmacy
SIGN UP AT
THEAPOTHECARYFARM.COM
TO JOIN THE FUN!

# HERBAL
## BLENDS



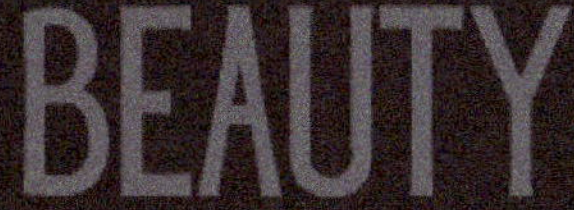

## BEAUTY

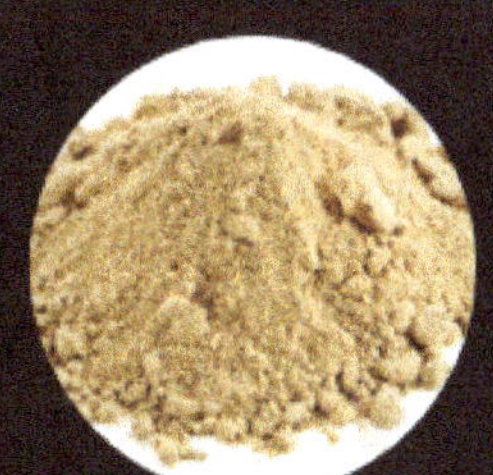

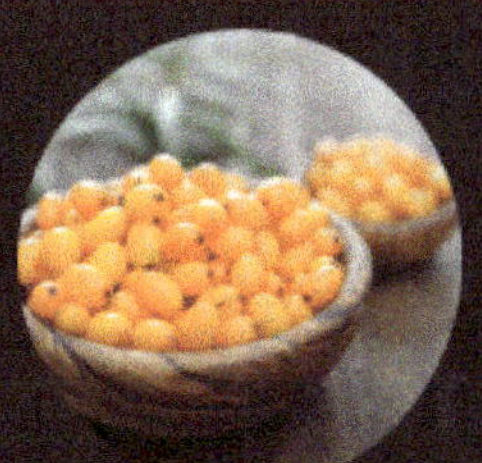

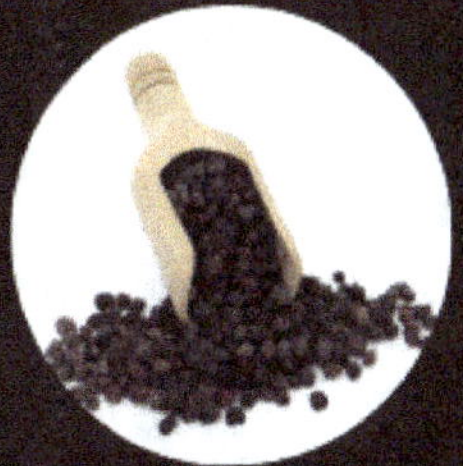

### ANTI-AGING BEAUTY TRIO

Better Than Botox -is a 3x plant based collagen blend, containing three of Mother Nature's most potent sources of skin food: Camu Camu, Sea Buckthorn and Schisandra Berry.

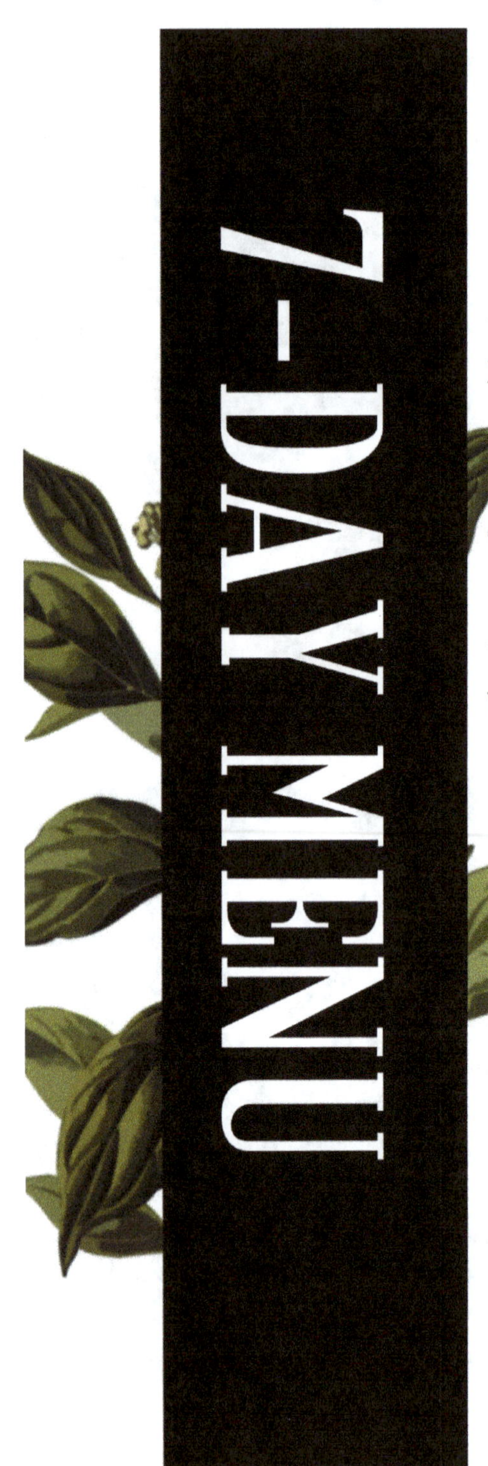

# 7-DAY MENU

| | Breakfast | Lunch | Dinner |
|---|---|---|---|
| **Monday** | Peanutbutter Overnight Oats | Lentil Stew | Thai Veggie Curry |
| **Tuesday** | Banana Pancakes | Thai Veggie Curry | Lentil Stew |
| **Wednesday** | Peanutbutter Overnight Oats | Lentil Stew | Thai Veggie Curry |

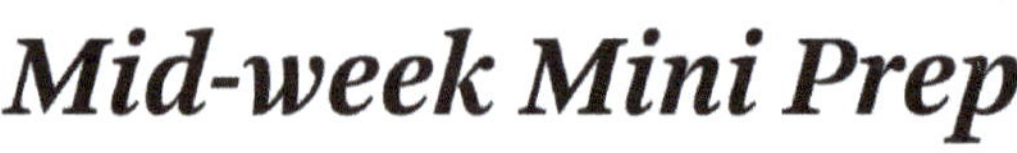

## *Mid-week Mini Prep*

| | Breakfast | Lunch | Dinner |
|---|---|---|---|
| **Thursday** | Banana Pancakes | Quinoa Powersalad | Buddha Bowl |
| **Friday** | Peanutbutter Overnight Oats | Buddha Bowl | Quinoa Power-salad |

# Grocery List

**This is for 1 person. If you cook for more people, multiply accordingly.**

## Fresh Produce

- 4 medium bananas
- your favorite berries (optional)
- 2 celery stalk
- 2 onions
- 2 leeks
- 4 cloves garlic
- 4 cups kale
- 2 large sweet potatoes
- 2 large white potatos
- 2 carrots
- 1 knob ginger
- 1 red bell pepper
- 1 jalapeno
- 1 pint grape tomatoes
- 4 scallions
- 1 bunch fresh cilantro
- 2 avocados
- 2 lemons
- 1 small cauliflower head
- 1 cup red cabbage

## Canned and Boxed

- 3.5 cups wholegrain oats
- 2.5 cups unsweetend almond milk (or other plant-based milk)
- 3 tbsp peanutbutter
- 3 tbsp chia seeds
- 2 cans brown lentils
- 2 cans chopped tomatoes
- 4 cups vegetable broth
- 1 can full-fat coconut milk
- 2 cans chickpeas
- 2 cups dry quinoa
- 3 tbsp peanuts (optional)
- 1 can sweet corn

*DON'T FORGET TO CHECK YOUR PANTRY!*

## Condiments and Spices

- 2 tablespoons extra virgin olive oil (optional)
- canola oil (optional)
- 1/2 teaspoon vanilla extract
- 1 teaspoon cumin
- 1 teaspoon cinnamon
- salt and pepper to taste
- 1 tbsp apple cider vinegar
- 1 tsp baking powder
- 1/4 tsp chili powder (optional)
- 1 tbsp soy sauce
- 2 tbsp tahini
- 2 tbsp red curry paste
- 3 tbsp maple syrup

## Equipments

- non-stick pan (if you avoid oil)
- blender
- glass jar (or sealable container)
- at least 3 other sealable containers

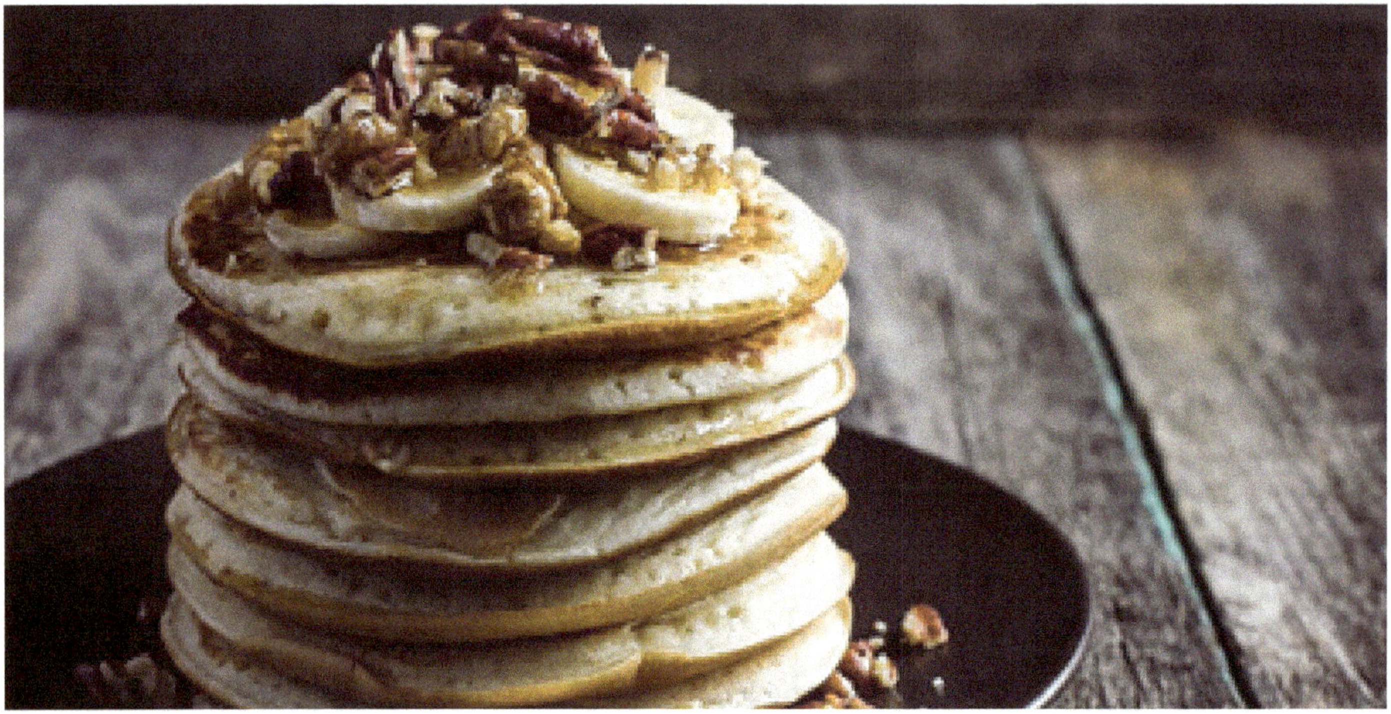

# Banana Pancakes

*3 Servings / 15 Minutes*

### Ingredients

1 1/2 cups oats
2 ripe bananas
1/2 cup almond milk
1 tsp cinnamon
1 tbsp apple cider vinegar
1 tsp baking powder
canola oil for frying (optional)

### Nutrition Facts

| | |
|---|---|
| Servings Per Recipe: | 3 |
| Serving Size: | 1 serving |
| Calories: | 460 |
| Total Fat: | 18 g |
| Saturated Fat: | 1.8 g |
| Cholesterol: | 0.0 mg |
| Sodium: | 291 mg |
| Potassium: | 691 mg |
| Total Carbohydrate: | 69 g |
| Dietary Fiber: | 9.6 g |
| Sugars: | 15.1 g |
| Protein: | 9.7 g |

### Instructions

♦ In a food processor, blend the oats until it has a flour like consistency.

♦ Add the bananas, milk, cinnamon and apple cider vinegar. Pulse until the batter is smooth. Let it sit for 10 minutes, then add the baking powder and blend until just incorporated.

♦ Cook the pancakes in a large pan on medium high heat in a non-stick pan or with a little oil until bubbles form on top. Flip and continue cooking until golden brown.

68%
TARGETS

35%
PROTEIN

56%
IRON

27%
CALCIUM

38%
VIT. E

129%
VIT. C

17%
SELENIUM

52%
OMEGA-3

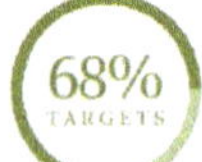

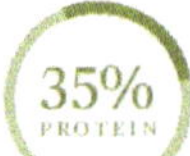

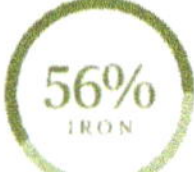

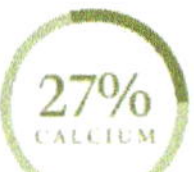

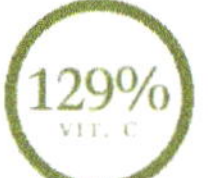

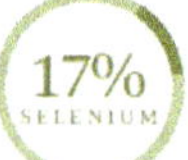

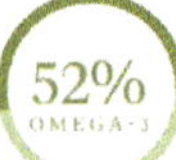

***Notes:***
***Serve (but don't store) with your favourite berries, nut butter or maple syrup. Delicious!***

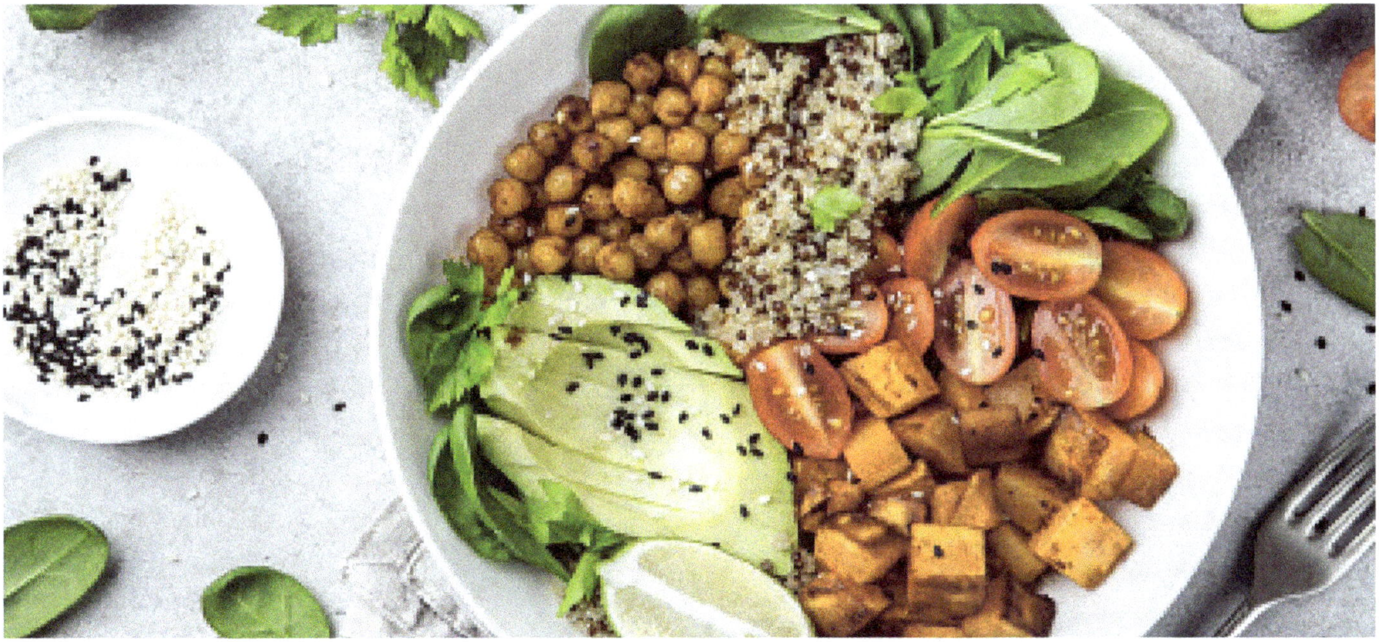

# Budhha Bowel

*2 Servings / 40 Minutes*

### Ingredients

1 sweet potato
1 can chickpeas
1 tbsp soy sauce
1 garlic
1 cup red cabbage
1/2 bunch of coriander
1 cup kale
1 avocado
2 tablespoons of tahini
1/2 lemon
2 cups cooked quinoa

### Nutrition Facts

| | |
|---|---|
| Servings Per Recipe: | 2 |
| Serving Size: | 1 serving |
| Calories: | 649 |
| Total Fat: | 24.9 g |
| Saturated Fat: | 3.3 g |
| Cholesterol: | 0.0 mg |
| Sodium: | 562 mg |
| Potassium: | 1460 mg |
| Total Carbohydrate: | 92.8 g |
| Dietary Fiber: | 21.7 g |
| Sugars: | 13.7 g |
| Protein: | 22.1 g |

### Instructions

♦ Preheat your oven to 180°C. Peel the sweet potatoes and cut into medium sized chunks. Put onto a roasting tray together with chickpeas, drizzle with olive oil and season with salt and pepper. Roast for 40 minutes until the potatoes are soft and the chickpeas crunchy.

♦ Thinly slice the cabbage. Slice the radishes and avocado, squeeze a little remaining lemon juice over the avocado to stop it going brown.

♦ Add your tahini to a bowl with the juice of half a lemon, a grated garlic clove, salt, pepper and olive oil. Add enough water to make a drizzalable dressing the tahini always seizes when you first add the lemon juice, keep adding water until it comes back together. Once thick and creamy, season with salt and pepper.

♦ Add your kale to a roasting tray. Season with salt and pepper. Drizzle over some olive oil. Mix together and roast for 10 mins until crispy

♦ Add your precooked quinoa to a large bowl. Then add all your various bits. Top with roasted kale, some coriander leaves and tahini dressing.

68%
TARGETS

35%
PROTEIN

56%
IRON

27%
CALCIUM

38%
VIT. E

129%
VIT. C

17%
SELENIUM

52%
OMEGA-3

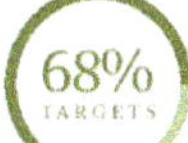

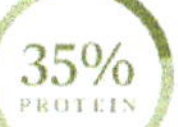

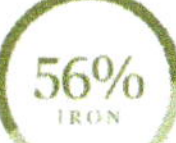

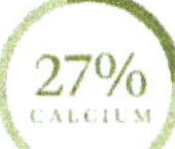

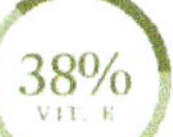

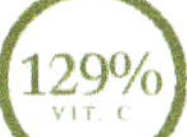

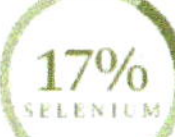

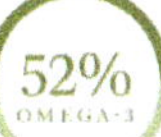

***Note:***
***Buddha Bowls are perfect for throwing together all of the leftovers at the end of the week! So feel free to adjust this recipe to your liking.***

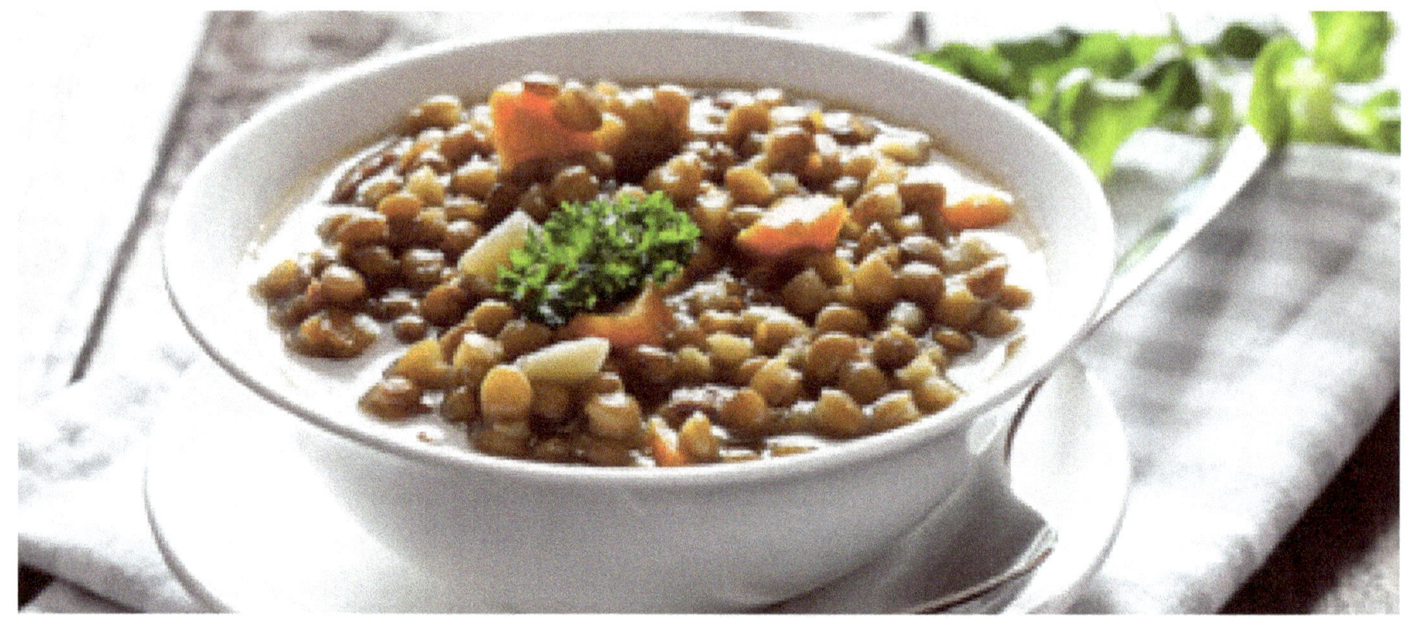

# Hearty Lentil Stew

*3 Servings / 45 Minutes*

**Ingredients**

2 large onions, chopped
2 tbsp canola oil
2 celery stalks, chopped
2 leeks, chopped
3 cloves garlic, minced
2 cans brown lentils
2 cups kale, chopped
2 large carrots, peeled and cut into large pieces
2 large potatoes, peeled and chopped into pieces
2 7-ounce cans chopped tomatoes
4 cups low-sodium vegetable broth
2 cups water
1 teapsoon cumin
dash of cinnamon
salt and pepper to taste

**Nutrition Facts**

| | |
|---|---|
| Servings Per Recipe: | 3 |
| Serving Size: | 1 serving |
| Calories: | 560 |
| Total Fat: | 8.5 g |
| Saturated Fat: | 0.9 g |
| Cholesterol: | 0.0 mg |
| Sodium: | 1650 mg |
| Potassium: | 2334 mg |
| Total Carbohydrate: | 105.4 g |
| Dietary Fiber: | 23.4 g |
| Sugars: | 17.5 g |
| Protein: | 24.4 g |

**Instructions**

♦ Heat the oil in a large pot or Dutch oven over medium heat.

♦ Add the onions, celery, and leeks and cook for about 4 to 5 minutes.

♦ Add the garlic and for another minute or two. Add the remaining ingredients

♦ Bring to a boil, then cover, and let simmer on medium-low heat for about 30 minutes or until lentils are tender.

68%
TARGETS

35%
PROTEIN

56%
IRON

27%
CALCIUM

38%
VIT. E

129%
VIT. C

17%
SELENIUM

52%
OMEGA-3

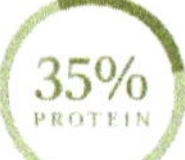

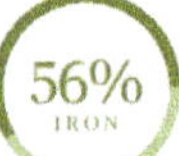

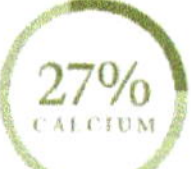

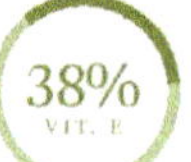

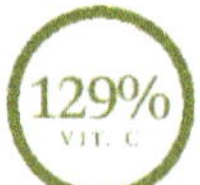

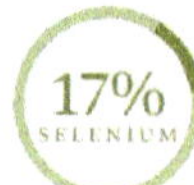

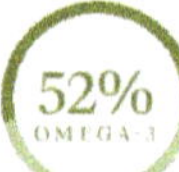

***Notes:***
***Dip in some whole-wheat bread to make it even more satisfying when the big hunger hits!***

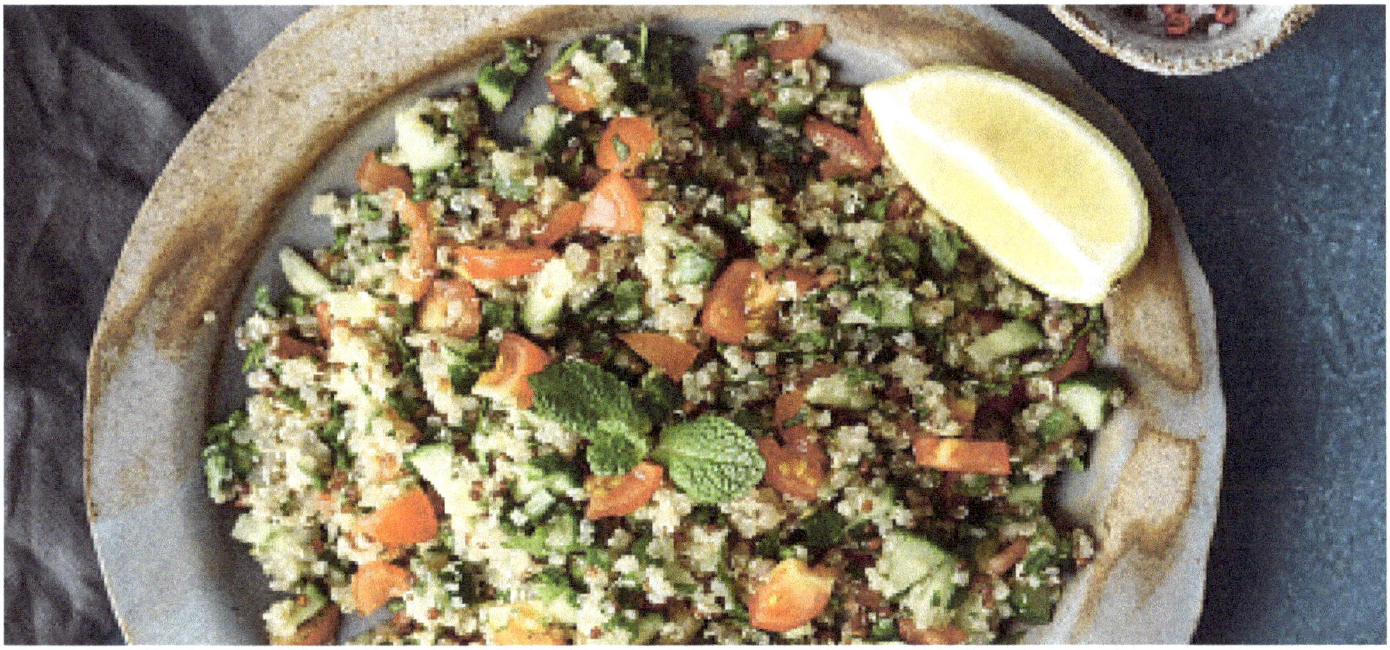

# Quinoa Powersalad

*2 Servings / 20 Minutes*

**Ingredients**

2 cups dry quinoa
1 red bell pepper, diced
1 jalapeño, finely chopped (optional)
1 cup of cooked corn
1 pint grape tomatoes, halved
4 fresh scallions, thinly sliced
1/2 cup fresh cilantro, roughly chopped
1 avocado, diced
Zest from 1/2 lemon
Dressing:
1/8 cup olive oil
1/2 lemon, juiced
1 garlic clove, minced
1/4 teaspoon cumin
1/4 teaspoon chili powder (optional)
1/4 teaspoon salt

**Nutrition Facts**

| | |
|---|---|
| Servings Per Recipe: | 2 |
| Calories: | 583 |
| Total Fat: | 29.2g |
| Saturated Fat: | 4 g |
| Cholesterol: | 0.0 mg |
| Sodium: | 499 mg |
| Potassium: | 1435 mg |
| Total Carbohydrate: | 74.5 g |
| Dietary Fiber: | 15.8 g |
| Sugars: | 15.2 g |
| Protein: | 14.6 g |

**Instructions**

- Add all of the dressing ingredients to a small bowl and whisk very well to combine. Set aside.
- Add half of the cooked (and cooled) quinoa to a large serving bowl. Add everything to the serving bowl with the quinoa, except the avocado. Toss very well to combine.
- Top with avocado and lime juice- You can also add another small handful or two of the fresh scallions and fresh cilantro. Salt and pepper to taste.
- Keep the salad and dressing in seperate containers and combine shortly before eating it.

43% TARGETS

19%
PROTEIN

27%
IRON

44%
CALCIUM

53%
VIT. E

9%
VIT. C

40%
SELENIUM

124%
OMEGA 3

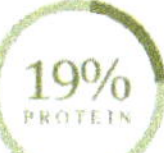

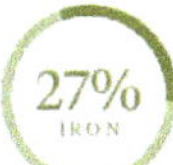

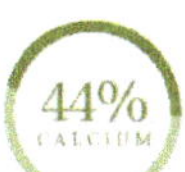

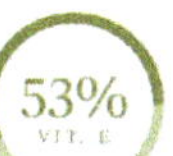

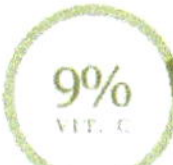

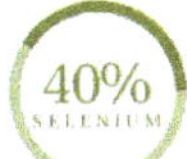

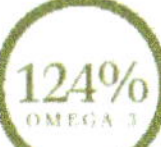

***Notes:***
***The lemon juice will keep the avocado from getting brown while sitting in the fridge.***
***It's important to keep salad and dressing seperated until the last moment to prevent it from getting soggy.***
***You can cook all of the dry quinoa at once and and use the leftovers for the buddha bowl.***

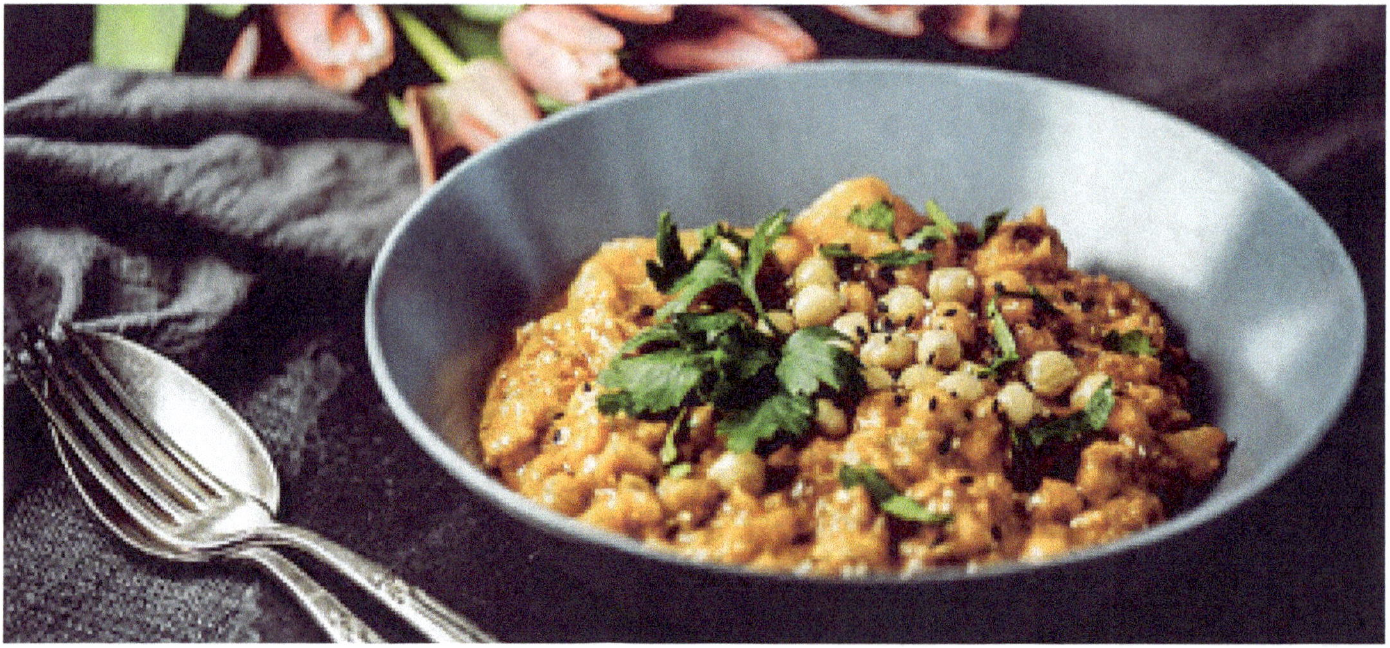

# Chickpea Curry

*3 Servings / 45 Minutes*

### Ingredients

1 tbsp canola cooking oil
1 large onion, sliced into half moons
1 garlic clove, minced
2 tsp grated ginger
4 tbsp red curry paste
1 can full fat coconut milk
1 tsp salt
2 cups sweet potatoes cut into bite-sized chunks
1 cup cauliflower florets
1 can chickpeas, drained and rinsed
1 cup kale

### Nutrition Facts

| | |
|---|---|
| Servings Per Recipe: | 3 |
| Serving Size: | 1 serving |
| Calories: | 449 |
| Total Fat: | 12.4 g |
| Saturated Fat: | 2.6 g |
| Cholesterol: | 0.0 mg |
| Sodium: | 2200 mg |
| Potassium: | 1545 mg |
| Total Carbohydrate: | 75.3 g |
| Dietary Fiber: | 17 g |
| Sugars: | 22.7 g |
| Protein: | 15.3 g |

### Instructions

♦ Heat oil in a large stock pot. Cook onions until fragrant, then add garlic and ginger. Cook for 1 minute until fragrant then add curry paste, cook stirring paste with the vegetables for 1 minute.

♦ Whisk in coconut milk. Add the salt.

♦ Then add the sweet potatoes. Allow to cook in the curry for 5-8 mins until tender.

♦ Then add the cauliflower, chickpeas and kale. Cook until heated through and tender about 5 mins more.

♦ Transfer to 3 containers along side of brown rice or quinoa.

43%
TARGETS

19%
PROTEIN

27%
IRON

44%
CALCIUM

53%
VIT. E

9%
VIT. C

40%
SELENIUM

124%
OMEGA-3

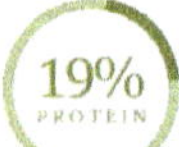

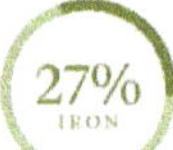

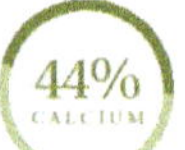

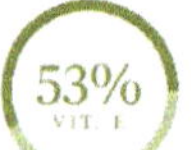

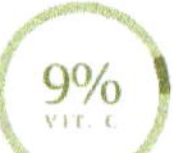

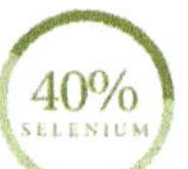

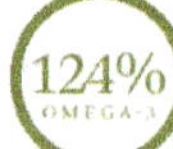

***Notes:***
***Delicious by itself or served with brown rice, quinoa, millet to make it even more satisfying.***

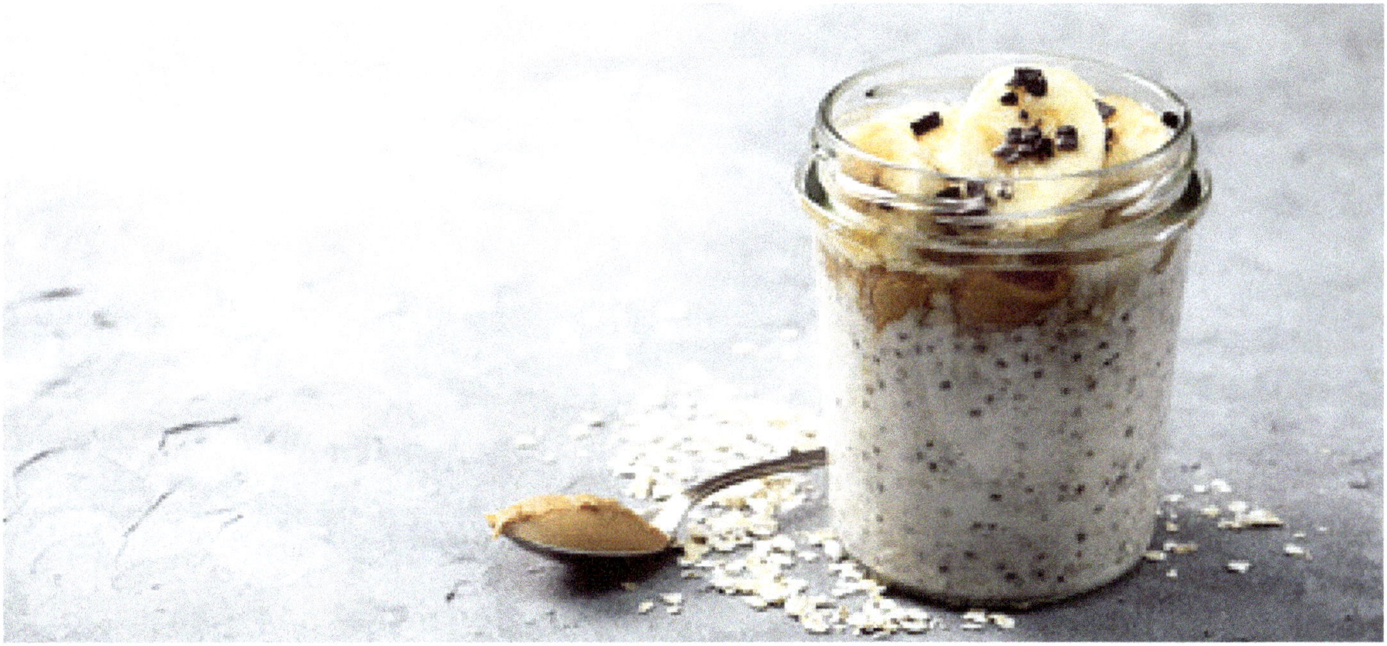

# Peanut Butter Overnight Oats

*3 Servings / 5 Minutes*

**Ingredients**

2 cups old fashioned oats
2 cups unsweetened almond milk
3 tbsp peanut butter
3 tbsp chia seeds
3 tbsp maple syrup
1 1/2 tsp vanilla extract
2 medium banana, sliced
2 tbsp peanuts, crushed

**Nutrition Facts**

| | |
|---|---|
| Servings Per Recipe: | 3 |
| Serving Size: | 1 serving |
| Calories: | 485 |
| Total Fat: | 16.6 g |
| Saturated Fat: | 2.7 g |
| Cholesterol: | 0.0 mg |
| Sodium: | 190 mg |
| Potassium: | 743 mg |
| Total Carbohydrate: | 73.9 g |
| Dietary Fiber: | 11.3 g |
| Sugars: | 24 g |
| Protein: | 13.6 g |

**Instructions**

♦ Combine oats, almond milk, peanut butter, chia seeds, syrup, and vanilla in a bowl. Mix well then transfer to sealable container (glass jars work well).

♦ Place in refrigerator.

♦ To serve, place a scoop of peanut butter oats in a bowl and top with sliced bananas and crushed peanuts.

43% TARGETS

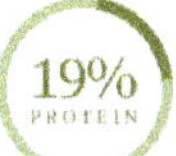

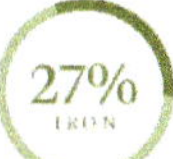

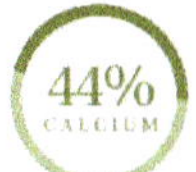

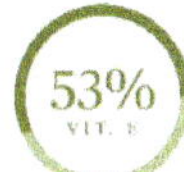

19%
PROTEIN

27%
IRON

44%
CALCIUM

53%
VIT. E

9% VIT. C

40%
SELENIUM

124%
OMEGA-3

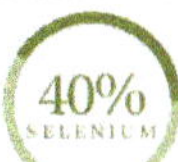

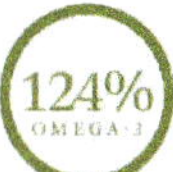

***Notes:***
***Can be stored for up to 5 days in the fridge.***
***They will continue to soften the longer they sit — which might be a bonus if you like your oatmeal on the super-creamy side***

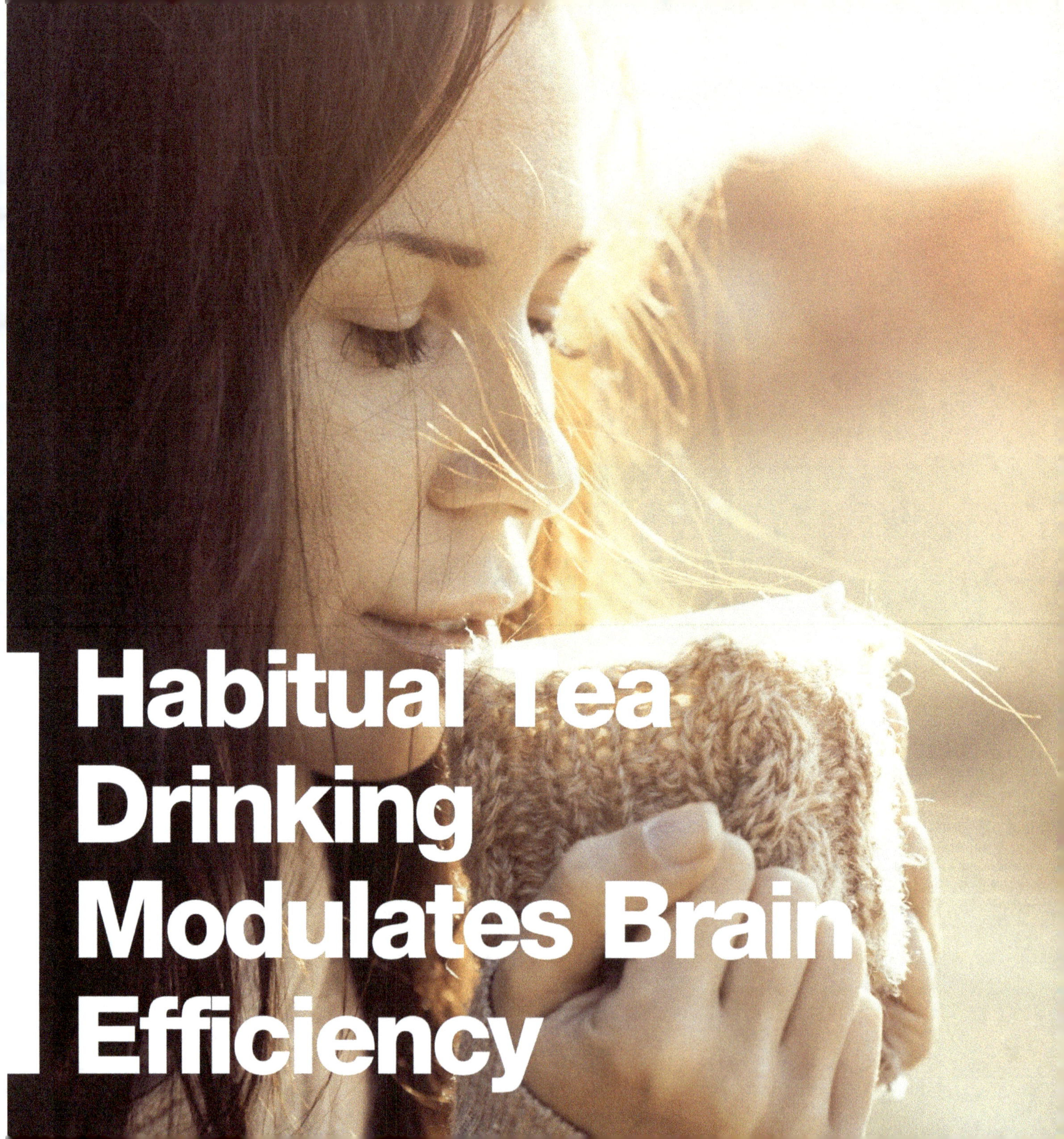

# Habitual Tea Drinking Modulates Brain Efficiency

**The researchers recruited healthy older participants to two groups according to their history of tea drinking frequency and investigated both functional and structural networks to reveal the role of tea drinking on brain organization.**

The suppression of hemispheric asymmetry in the structural connectivity network was observed as a result of tea drinking.

The authors did not observe any significant effects of tea drinking on the hemispheric asymmetry of the functional connectivity network.

> Dr. Junhua Li and Dr. Lei Feng said, "Tea has been a popular beverage since antiquity, with records referring to consumption dating back to the dynasty of Shen Nong (approximately 2700 BC) in China."

Tea is consumed in diverse ways, with brewed tea and products with a tea ingredient extremely prevalent in Asia, especially in China and Japan.

Although individual constituents of tea have been related to the roles of maintaining cognitive abilities and preventing cognitive decline, a study with behavioural and neurophysiological measures showed that there was a degraded effect or no effect when a constituent was administered alone and a significant effect was observed only when constituents were combined.

The superior effect of the constituent combination was also demonstrated in a comparative experiment that suggested that tea itself should be administered instead of tea extracts; a review of tea effects on the prevention of Alzheimers disease, found that the neuroprotective role of herbal tea was apparent in eight out of nine studies.

It is worth noting that the majority of studies thus far have evaluated tea effects from the perspective of neurocognitive and neuropsychological measures, with direct measurement of brain structure or function less-well represented in the extant literature.

These studies focusing on brain regional alterations did not ascertain tea effects on interregional interactions at the level of the entire brain.

> The Li/Feng Research team concluded, "In summary, our study comprehensively investigated the effects of tea drinking on brain connectivity at both global and regional scales using multi-modal imaging data and provided the first compelling evidence that tea drinking positively contributes to brain structure making network organization more efficient."

# HERBAL BLENDS

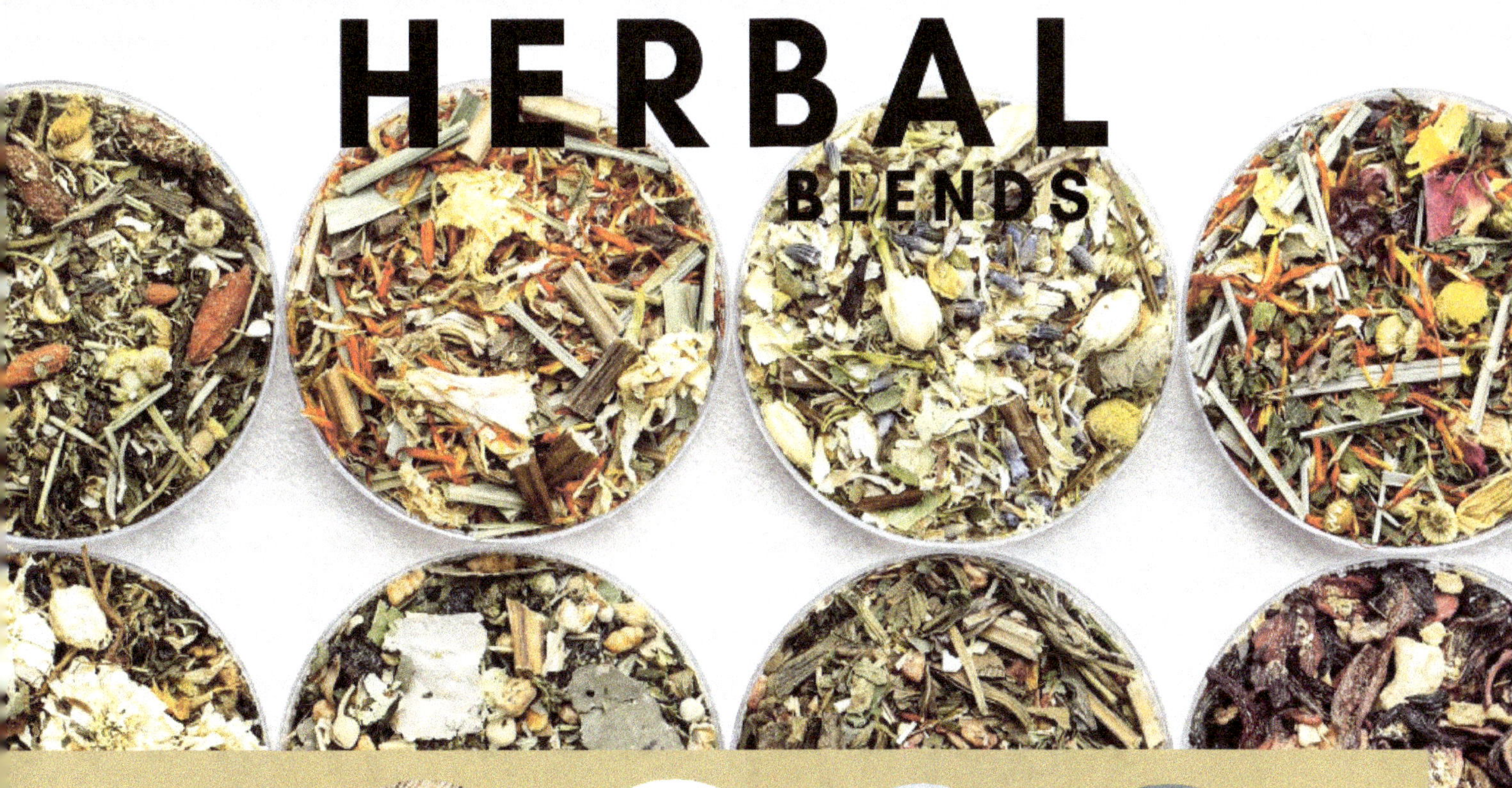

## GLOW

PAIRS WELL WITH: KOMBUCHA, FRUIT SMOOTHIES, AND LIME + MINT WATER.

One of the major factors in rapid aging and the deterioration of our skin is inflammation. Glow Blend is a unique anti-inflammatory combination of cooling yin properties will cater to your complexion's warm-weather needs: Goji Berry, Reishi mushroom, He Shou Wu, Maca Root, Brand Rice

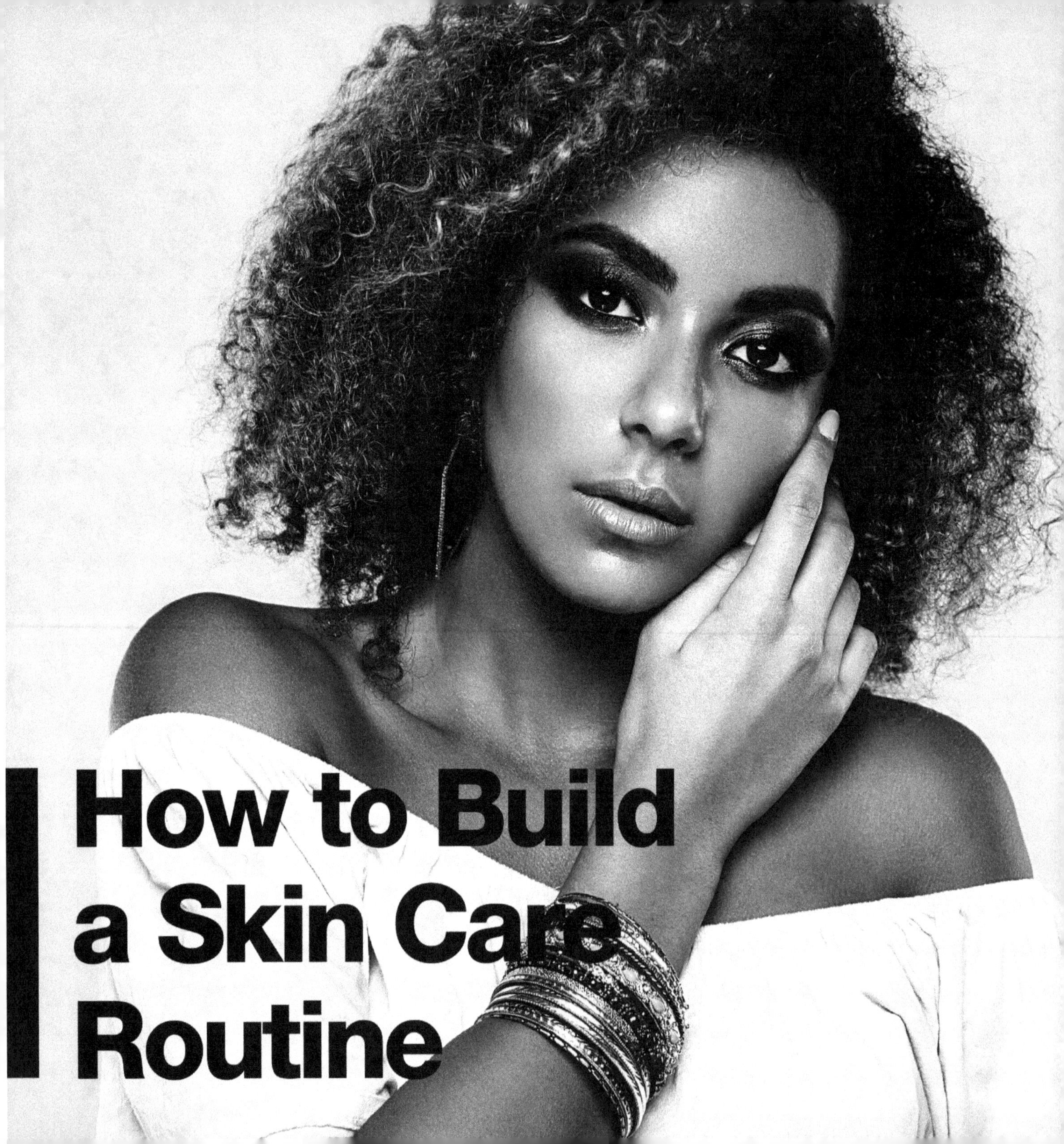

# How to Build a Skin Care Routine

Great skin is not simply a matter of DNA — your daily habits, in fact, have a big impact on what you see in the mirror. But depending on which product reviews you read or doctors you consult, there is a dizzying number of opinions on everything from how to moisturize to how to protect yourself from UV rays. Ultimately, caring for your skin is simply personal. Here's what you should keep in mind to sort through all the noise.

## Three Main Steps

Think of your skin-care routine as consisting of three main steps:

- Cleansing — Washing your face.
- Toning — Balancing the skin.
- Moisturizing — Hydrating and softening the skin.

The goal of any skin-care routine is to tune up your complexion so it's functioning at its best, and also troubleshoot or target any areas you want to work on. "Beauty routines are an opportunity to notice changes within yourself," says the San Francisco skin-care specialist Kristina Holey. As your skin needs shifts with age, so will your products. Still, she adds, "it's not about creating perfection." Allow these three steps to become your daily ritual that fortifies your skin and grounds your day.

## Give it Time

The science behind skin-care products has come a long way but there's still no such thing as an instant fix — you need time to reap the benefits, says Dr. Rachel Nazarian, a Manhattan dermatologist at Schweiger Dermatology Group. "Results are only seen through consistent use," she explains. Generally, aim to use a product over at least six weeks, once or twice daily, to notice a difference.

## Tip:

With any skin-care product, apply in order of consistency — from thinnest to thickest. For example, cleanser, toner (if you use it), serum, and then moisturizer.

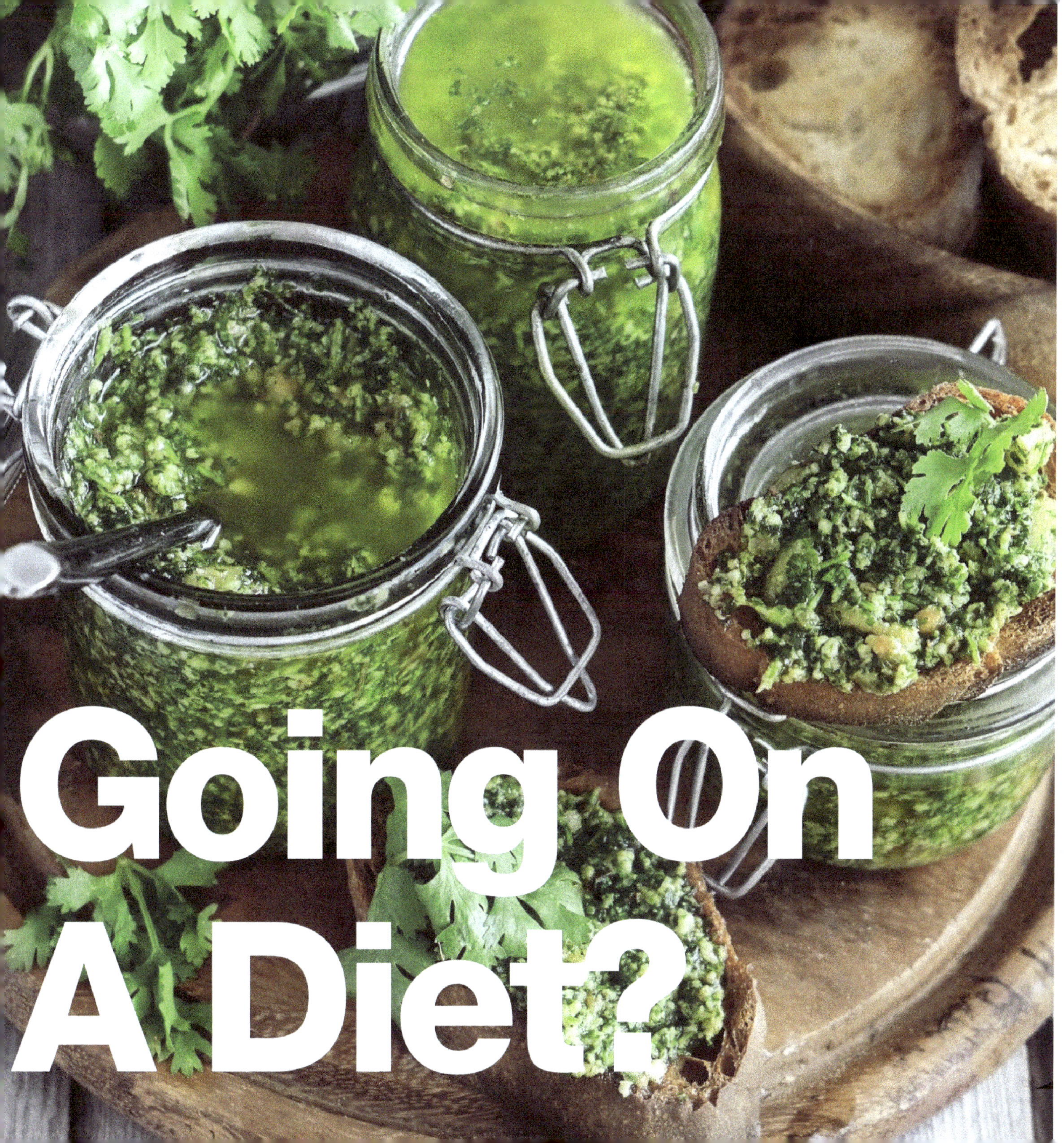

# Going On A Diet?

## We explain how dieting can affect your skin

A healthy, glowing complexion says a lot about your skin and your diet. The condition of our skin reflects what we eat and highlights the importance of looking after yourself from the inside out. Food is fuel and our bodies function best when we provide it with healthy, balanced and nutritious food.

Whilst many of us are conscious about our food intake when it comes to our waistlines, a healthy skin diet is also hugely important when it comes to getting gorgeous, healthy, glowing skin.

For those making the decision to change their diet, whether it is to lose weight or to make healthier food choices, it's important to be aware of the effect it may have on your skin.

## How certain foods can affect your skin:

A diet which consists of highly processed food, ready meals and refined carbohydrates can over time cause a mild inflammation in the body and aggravate skin problems such as acne1.

Whilst most of us know that an unhealthy diet is detrimental to our skin, did you know that diet plays a part in fighting the effects of sun (UV rays) damage on our skin? Exposure to UV rays promotes the formation of free radicals which can cause damage to components of our skin that gives it its structure and firmness such as elastin and collagen. Over a period of time, this can result in more prominent fine lines and wrinkles!

So, how does this link to your diet? Eating antioxidants-rich foods, such as colourful fruit and vegetables, helps to fight free radicals and some studies have shown that they can help improve skin texture2.

## Key food groups to be aware of which improve your skin – and which to avoid:

Fish is a brilliant source of protein (essential for collagen and elastin production keeping your skin supple) and contains omega-3 fatty acids known for promoting skin health and reducing inflammation.

Richly coloured orange or red fruit and vegetables get much of their colour from compounds called carotenoids, some of which can be converted into Vitamin A, which is essential for skin cell reproduction. They are also a great source of Vitamin C, which is essential for manufacturing collagen and both carotenoids and Vitamin C are antioxidants, helping to fight free radicals which may cause damage to our skin and cause premature signs of ageing 3,4.

Avoid refined carbs and sugars –these include sweets, white bread, pastries, white rice, sugary drinks and many breakfast cereals. Replace these foods with 'good carbs' such as healthy vegetables, whole grains and the wrinkle-fighting antioxidants found in fruits which have a lower glycemic index – in turn, reduce the overall carbohydrate load in your diet3.

Whilst on a diet, it is essential that your body gets enough water. Staying hydrated is very important in order for nutrients to reach your skin cells. Avoid sugary drinks and enjoy water or green tea which is known to be a brilliant source of antioxidants.

The healthier the diet choices you make, the more it shows in your skin.

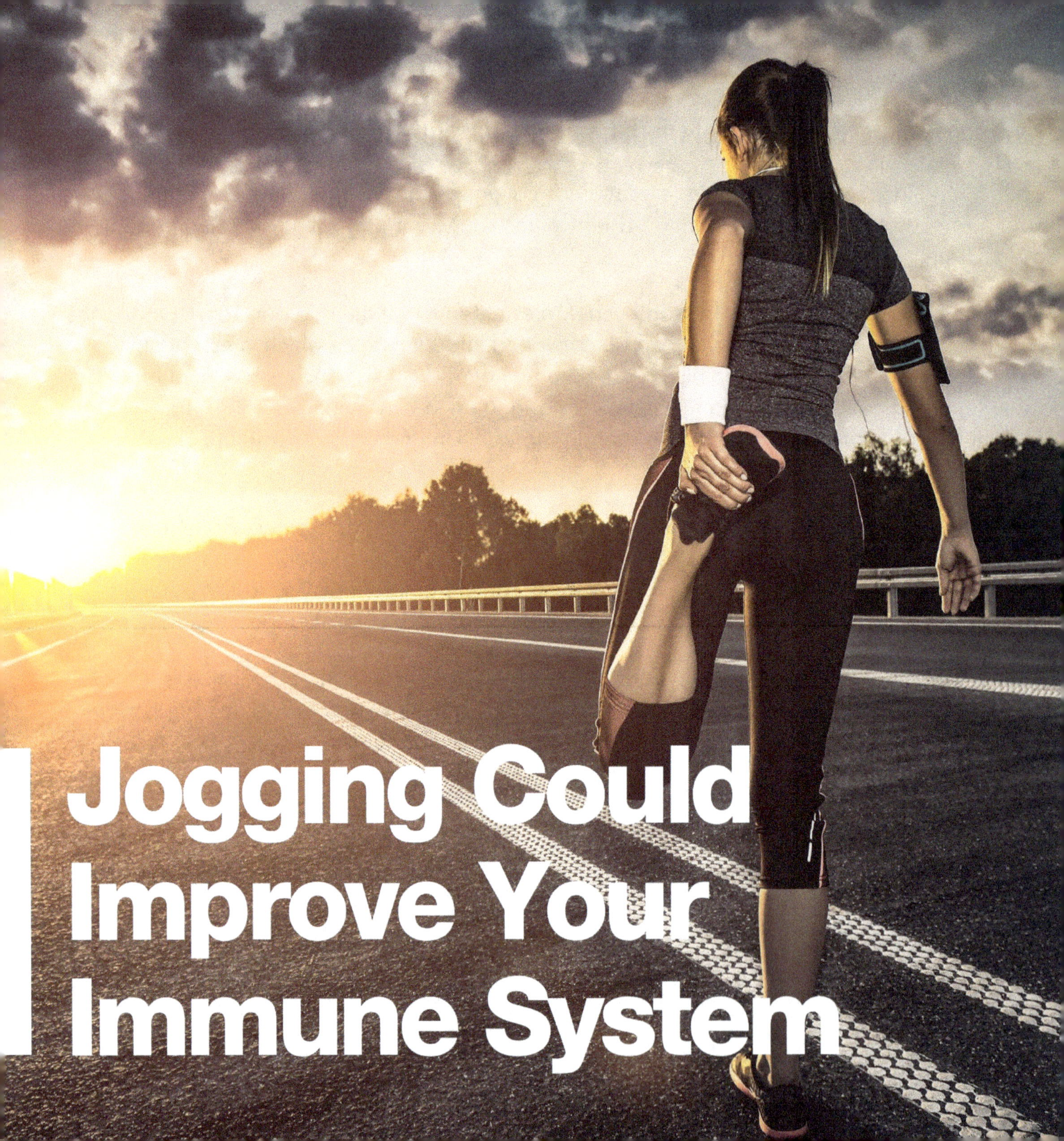

# Jogging Could Improve Your Immune System

If going for a jog every once in a while is good for you — and it is — then going jogging every day packs a whole world of potential benefits, from faster weight loss (or maintaining a healthy weight) to improved mood, more energy and lower risk of chronic diseases. You should, however, be alert to the possibility of overtraining, and the effects of repeated high-impact exercise on your body.

## The Benefits of Jogging Regularly

Health.gov's Dietary Guidelines for Americans recommends that adults should get at least 150 minutes of moderate intensity aerobic activity each week. If you go for a half-hour jog every day, that's enough to meet — and even beat — this requirement.

## Tip

The Dietary Guidelines also notes that doubling the amount of cardio exercise to 300 minutes of moderate exertion each week yields even more extensive health benefits.

So, what's on the menu for "better health through exercise"? The well-researched benefits of jogging and other cardiovascular exercise include:

- Weight loss
- Increased stamina
- A stronger immune system
- Decreased risk of chronic diseases, including obesity, heart disease, hypertension, type 2 diabetes and some cancers
- Help managing chronic conditions and improving quality of life
- An improved cholesterol profile
- A natural mood boost

## Weight Bearing and Impact

Jogging is also a weight-bearing activity that can help you build and maintain strong bones in your lower body, as long as your bones, joints and muscles can handle the repeated impact of each footfall. If you know you have weakened bones or any other condition that might affect your ability to withstand a relatively high-impact exercise, speak to your doctor before jogging every day.

Some of the steps you can take to mitigate the impact of jogging include:

- Wear supportive, well-cushioned footwear.
- Run on softer surfaces — such as dirt or wood chips — instead of pavement or cement.
- Warm up and stretch before you jog; then cool down and stretch after, to reduce your risk of injury.

You can also try "water jogging" in the pool, with a flotation belt to keep you above water. This gives you all the cardiovascular benefits of jogging, with none of the impact on your bones and joints.

Read more: The 8 Best Stretches to Do Before Running

## A Note for Beginners

If you're new to exercising, or new to a particular type of exercise, it's typical at first to develop some soreness — so that is one of the effects you might experience when you first start jogging. The good news is that this type of muscle soreness typically fades within a few days, and as your body adapts to the new exercise the soreness is less likely to come back.

While a little soreness is typical, it doesn't have to be intense. You can minimize the soreness by taking it relatively easy on your first jogs and gradually working up to longer distances or faster outings. While jumping straight into a long, fast jog can be exciting and make you feel like you've accomplished something big, it might also leave you too sore to go jogging for several days. So the slow and steady approach, while less dramatic, is more satisfying in the long run.

## Different Types of Jogging

Even if you really love jogging, doing the same thing every single day might eventually start to feel boring. And if you don't vary the challenges you present your body, you might also hit a fitness or weight-loss plateau.

You can still go jogging every day, but don't be shy about mixing up your jogging workouts every so often to present new challenges or at least a new experience:

- Choose different routes — both for the scenery and for the challenge of new terrain.
- Jog up hills or, for a real thigh-burner, jog down those hills.
- Go "trail jogging" on fun hiking or running trails.
- Hit the gym and "jog" on an elliptical trainer during rainy days.

You can also add variety to your jogs by switching up your speed. Go for a shorter, faster jog on days when you have limited time, or take it easy and go for a longer, moderate-pace jog when you have more time to work with.

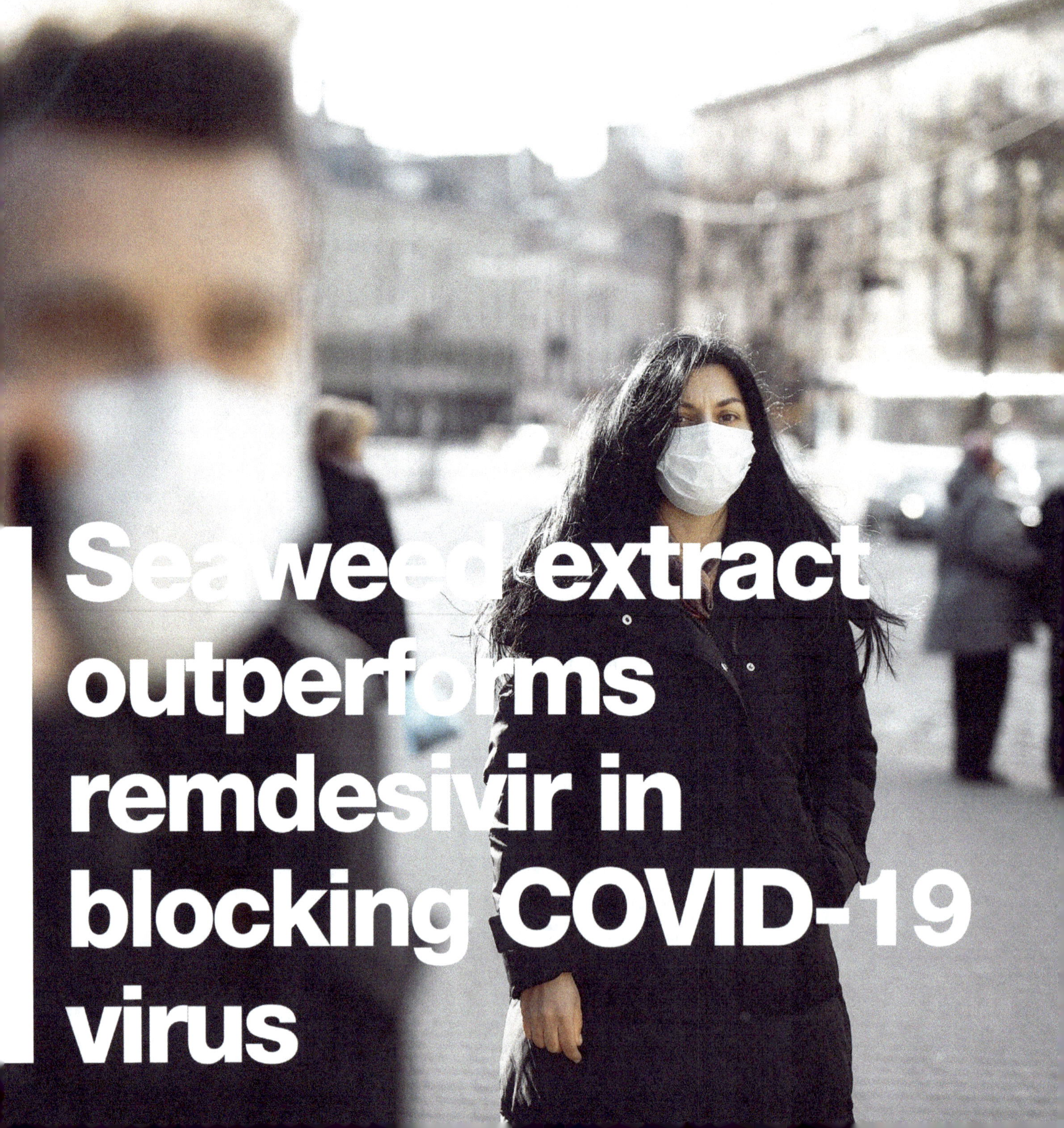

# Seaweed extract outperforms remdesivir in blocking COVID-19 virus

Heparin, a common anitcoagulent, could also form basis of a viral trap for SARS-CoV-2

In a test of antiviral effectiveness against the virus that causes COVID-19, an extract from edible seaweeds substantially outperformed remdesivir, the current standard antiviral used to combat the disease. Heparin, a common blood thinner, and a heparin variant stripped of its anticoagulant properties, performed on par with remdesivir in inhibiting SARS-CoV-2 infection in mammalian cells.

Published online today in Cell Discovery, the research is the latest example of a decoy strategy researchers from the Center for Biotechnology and Interdisciplinary Studies (CBIS) at Rensselear Polytechnic Institute are developing against viruses like the novel coronavirus that spawned the current global health crisis.

The spike protein on the surface of SARS-CoV-2 latches onto the ACE-2 receptor, a molecule on the surface of human cells. Once secured, the virus inserts its own genetic material into the cell, hijacking the cellular machinery to produce replica viruses. But the virus could just as easily be persuaded to lock onto a decoy molecule that offers a similar fit. The neutralized virus would be trapped and eventually degrade naturally.

Previous research has shown this decoy technique works in trapping other viruses, including dengue, Zika, and influenza A.

> "We're learning how to block viral infection, and that is knowledge we are going to need if we want to rapidly confront pandemics," said Jonathan Dordick, the lead researcher and a professor of chemical and biological engineering at Rensselaer Polytechnic Institute. "The reality is that we don't have great antivirals. To protect ourselves against future pandemics, we are going to need an arsenal of approaches that we can quickly adapt to emerging viruses."

The Cell Discovery paper tests antiviral activity in three variants of heparin (heparin, trisulfated heparin, and a non-anticoagulant low molecular weight heparin) and two fucoidans (RPI-27 and RPI-28) extracted from seaweed. All five compounds are long chains specific receptor on the cell surface.

"It's a very complicated mechanism that we quite frankly don't know all the details about, but we're getting more information," said Dordick. "One thing that's become clear with this study is that the larger the molecule, the better the fit. The more successful compounds are the larger sulfated polysaccharides that offer a greater number of sites on the molecules to trap the virus."

Molecular modeling based on the binding study revealed sites on the spike protein where the heparin was able to interact, raising the prospects for similar sulfated polysaccharides.

"This exciting research by Professors Dordick and Linhardt is among several ongoing research efforts at CBIS, as well as elsewhere at Rensselaer, to tackle the challenges of the COVID-19 pandemic through novel therapeutic approaches and the repurposing of existing drugs," said CBIS Director Deepak Vashishth.

"Sulfated polysaccharides effectively inhibit SARS-CoV-2 in vitro" was published in Cell Discovery with the support of the National Research Foundation of Korea. At Rensselaer, Dordick and Linhardt were joined in the research by Paul S. Kwon, Seok-Joon Kwon, Weihua Jin, Fuming Zhang, and Keith Fraser, and by researchers at the Korea Research Institute of Bioscience and Biotechnology in Cheongju, Republic of Korea, and Zhejiang University of Technology in Hangzhou, China.

# HERBAL BLENDS

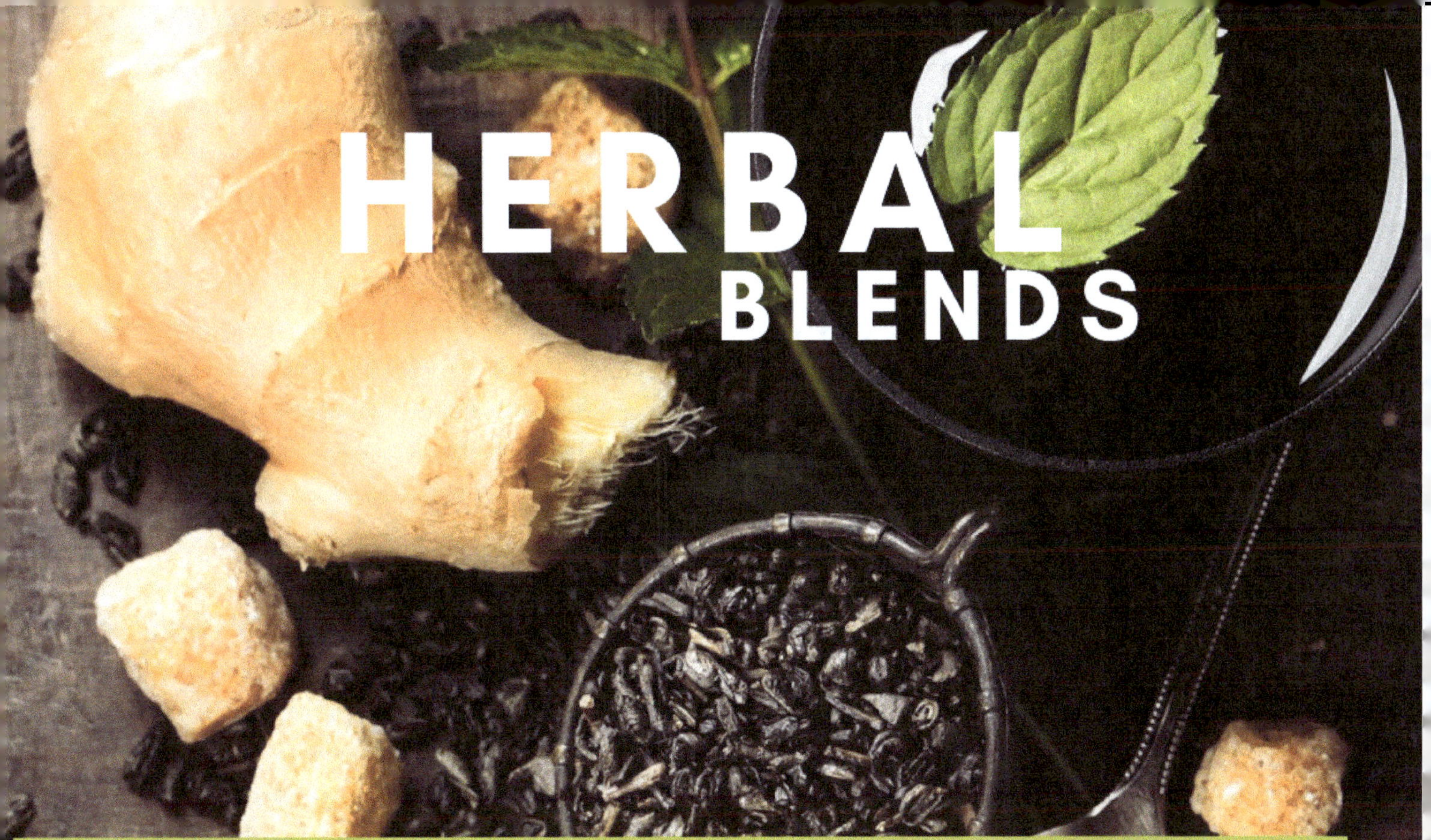

## IMMUNITY

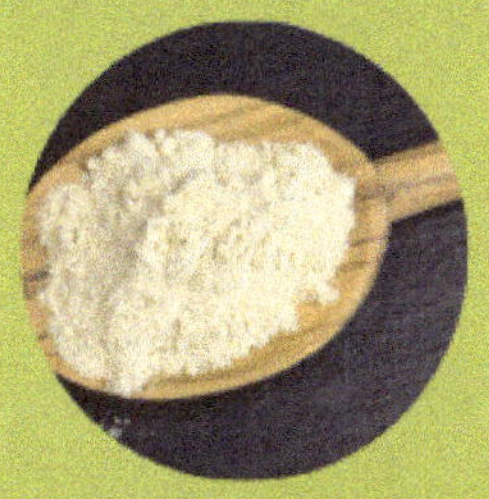

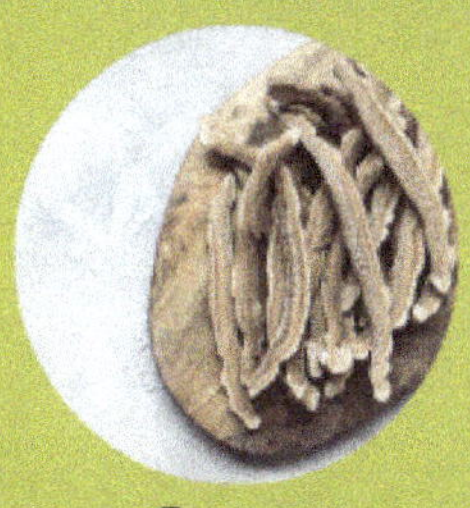

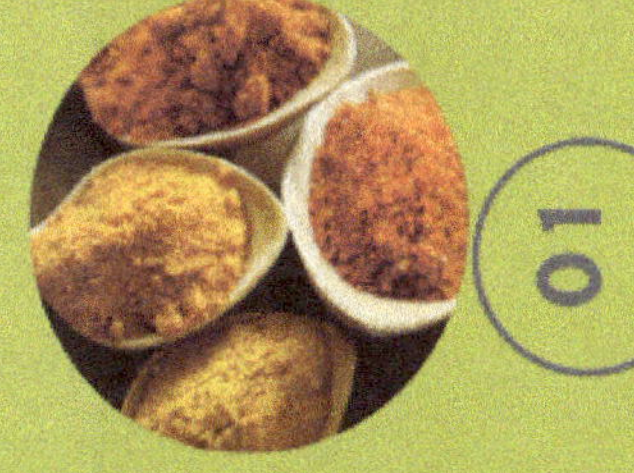

01

PAIRS WELL WITH: Coconut water, fruit smoothies, and lavender tea.

This Immunity trio includes two of our most popular Signature Blends and Reishi Mushroom. These powerful ingredients promote a heathy mind-body balance by boosting our immune system to protect our bodies from within. Reishi Mushroom and Ashwagandha Root

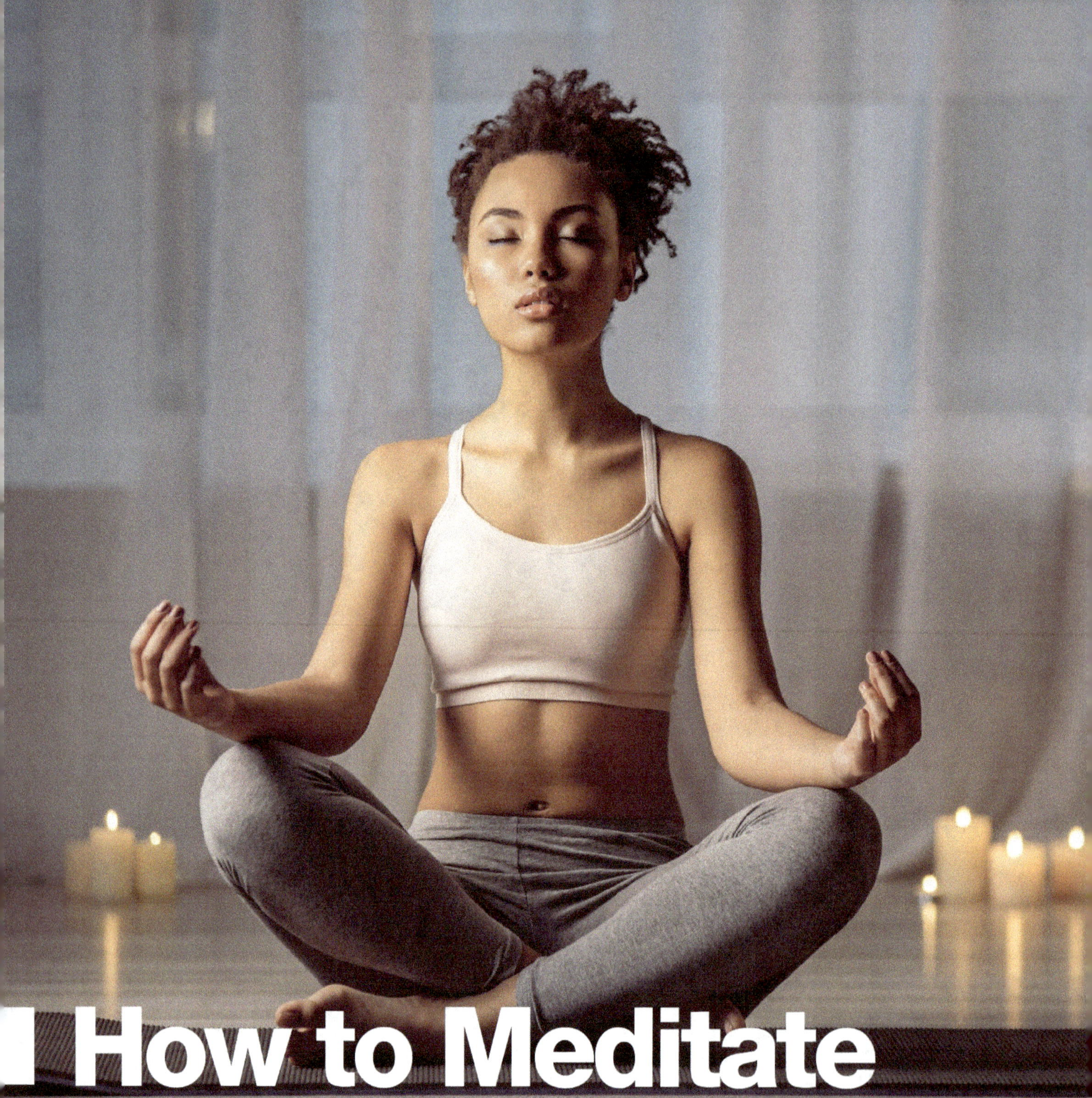

# How to Meditate

Meditation is a simple practice available to all, which can reduce stress, increase calmness and clarity and promote happiness. Learning how to meditate is straightforward, and the benefits can come quickly. Here, we offer basic tips to get you started on a path toward greater equanimity, acceptance and joy. Take a deep breath, and get ready to relax.

## Meditation Exercises

Find a comfortable spot and get ready to relax.

## The Basics

Setting aside time for formal meditation is an important way to establish a routine and get comfortable with the practice. Even just a few minutes a day can make a big difference.

> "Some people complain about taking time out of their day," said Atman Smith, who teaches meditation to underserved communities in Baltimore. "Practice is important though. It's a tool you can use to bring yourself back to the present in stressful situations."

But we shouldn't stop being mindful when we stop meditating. "The purpose of mindfulness meditation is to become mindful throughout all parts of our life, so that we're awake, present and openhearted in everything we do," said Tara Brach, a popular meditation teacher based near Washington, D.C. "Not just when we're sitting on the cushion."

Mindfulness meditation isn't about letting your thoughts wander. But it isn't about trying to empty your mind, either. Instead, the practice involves paying close attention to the present moment — especially our own thoughts, emotions and sensations — whatever it is that's happening.

In addition to basic meditation instructions, we've compiled guided meditations for a few popular exercises including the body scan, walking meditation and mindful eating.

"Each of the applied mindfulness practices brings alive an experience that might otherwise be more automatic," said Ms. Brach.

Though meditating on your own is an essential part of a complete practice, the steady guidance of an experienced teacher can be invaluable, especially as you're getting started. Our minds wander so easily, and the clear instructions of a teacher can help bring us back to the present moment.

## When the Mind Wanders

It's inevitable: During meditation, your mind will roam. You may notice other sensations in the body, things happening around you, or just get lost in thought, daydreaming about the past or present, possibly judging yourself or others.

There's nothing wrong with this — thinking is just as natural as breathing. "It's the natural conditioning of the mind to wander," said Ms. Brach.

When this happens, simply notice what it is you were thinking about or what was distracting you, then take a moment and pause.

You don't need to pull your attention right back to the breath. Instead, let go of whatever it was you were thinking about, reopen your attention, then gently return your awareness to the breath, being present for each inhalation and exhalation.

"Don't just drag the mind back to the breath," said Ms. Brach. "Instead reopen the attention, then gently come and land again."

After a few breaths, invariably, the mind will wander again. Don't beat yourself up about this. It's natural. What's important is how we respond when it happens. Simply acknowledge whatever it is you were thinking of — without ascribing too much judgment to it, without letting it carry you away — and take a moment to come back to the present, and resume your meditation.

"Where we build our skill is in the practice of coming back," said Ms. Brach. "Coming back again and again. Notice it — thinking — and then pause, and then come back to the present moment."

## Mindfulness Meditation Practices

You can practice mindfulness meditation on your own anytime and anywhere. But listening to basic guided meditations can also be helpful, especially when getting started. Instructions from an experienced teacher can help remind us to come back to the present moment, let go of distracting thoughts and not be so hard on ourselves.

Here are four guided meditations you can listen to that will help you remain in the present moment. Choose the one that's the right length for you:

One minute is a great place to start but also good if you simply don't have a lot of time. If you're more experienced or ready for an extended mindfulness session, try the 10- or 15-minute sessions. You can download these tracks and listen to them when you're ready to meditate.

## Body Scan

Instead of training your attention on the breath, as is the case in basic mindfulness meditation, the body scan involves systematically focusing on different sensations and areas, from the head to the toes.

Start at the top of your head. Slowly and deliberately, bring your attention to the surface of your skin, one inch at a time. See if you can feel your scalp, your ears, your eyelids and your nose. Continue in this manner, moving across the face, over the ears, down the neck and shoulders and all the way down to your toes.

At first, it might seem as if you don't feel anything at all. But as you progress, you might begin to notice a whole world of new sensations. Some of the feelings might be pleasant, a gentle warmth, a comfortable weight. Some feelings might be neutral — tingling or itching.

And some might be unpleasant. Your feet might feel soreness somewhere.

Whatever the sensation is, just note it. If you need to move to relieve real pain, do so. But try not to react — labeling the experience good or bad — even if it's unpleasant. Instead, just acknowledge what it is you're feeling, and continue with the body scan. And of course, if you realize your mind has wandered, simply note the thought, and return your attention to the body.

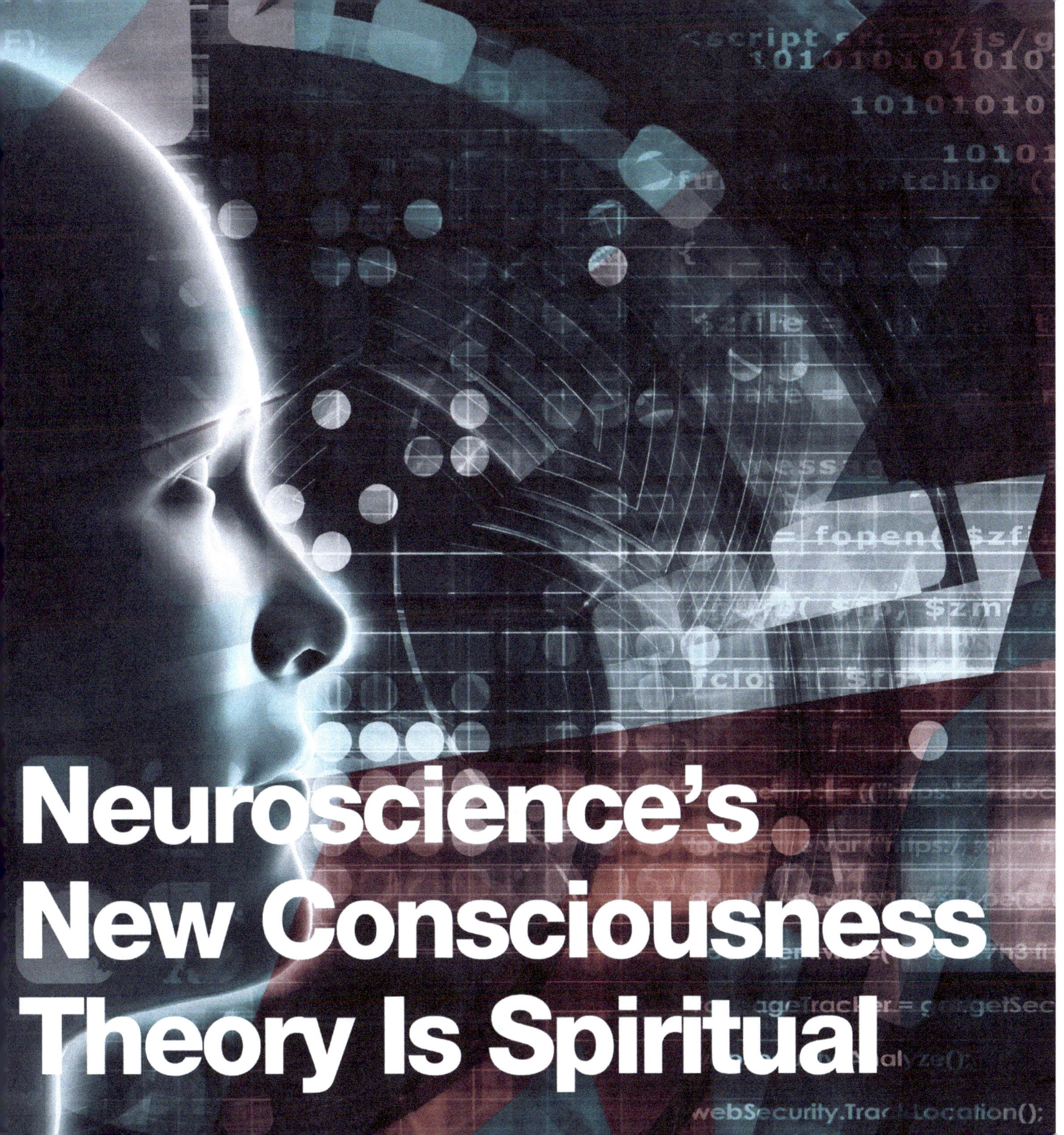

# Neuroscience's New Consciousness Theory Is Spiritual

Integrated Information Theory suggests that experience arises from information.

"Science is not only compatible with spirituality; it is a profound source of spirituality" -Carl Sagan

It appears that we are approaching a unique time in the history of man and science where empirical measures and deductive reasoning can actually inform us spiritually. Integrated Information Theory (IIT)—put forth by neuroscientists Giulio Tononi and Christof Koch—is a new framework that describes a way to experimentally measure the extent to which a system is conscious.

As such, it has the potential to answer questions that once seemed impossible, like "which is more conscious, a bat or a beetle?" Furthermore, the theory posits that any system that processes and integrates information, be it organic or inorganic, experiences the world subjectively to some degree. Plants, smartphones, the Internet—even protons—are all examples of such systems. The result is a cosmos composed of a sentient fabric. But before getting into the bizarreness of all that, let's talk a little about how we got to this point.

## The decline and demise of the mystical

As more of the natural world is described objectively and empirically, belief in the existence of anything that defies current scientific explanation is fading at a faster rate than ever before. The majority of college-educated individuals no longer accept the supernatural and magical accounts of physical processes given by religious holy books. Nor do they believe in the actuality of mystical realms beyond life that offer eternal bliss or infinite punishment for the "souls" of righteous or evil men.

This is because modern science has achieved impeccable performance when it comes to explaining phenomena previously thought to be unexplainable. In this day and age, we have complete scientific descriptions of virtually everything. We understand what gives rise to vacuous black holes and their spacetime geometries. We know how new species of life can evolve and the statistical rules that govern such processes. We even have a pretty good understanding of the exact moment in which the universe, and thus of all reality, came into existence! But no serious and informed scientist will tell you that at present we fully understand the thing each of us knows best. That is, our own consciousness.

## One of science's last greatest mysteries

Although we've come along way since the time of Descartes, who postulated that consciousness was actually some immaterial spirit not subject to physical law, we still don't have a complete and satisfactory account of the science underlying experience. We simply don't know how to quantify it. And if we can't do that, how do we know whether those non-human life forms that are unable to communicate with us are also conscious? Does it feel like anything to be a cat? Most will probably agree that it does, but how about a ladybug? If so, how can we know which life forms are more conscious than others? Do animals that show impressively intelligent behavior and elaborate memory, like dolphins or crows, experience the world in a unified conscious fashion as we do? These questions are almost impossible to answer without a way to measure consciousness. Fortunately, a neuroscientific theory that has been gaining popular acceptance aims to do just that.

## Integrated Information Theory to the Rescue

Integrated Information Theory (IIT), which has become quite a hot topic in contemporary neuroscience, claims to provide a precise way to measure consciousness and express the phenomenon in purely mathematical terms. The theory was put forth by psychiatrist and neuroscientist Giulio Tononi, and has attracted some highly regarded names in the science community. One such name is Christof Koch, Chief Scientific Officer at the Allen Institute for Brain Science, who now champions the idea along with Tononi. Koch may be best-known for bringing consciousness research into the mainstream of neuroscience through his long-term collaboration with the late DNA co-discoverer Francis Crick. Now Tononi and Koch are actively researching the theory along with an increasing number of scientists, some from outside the field of neuroscience like esteemed physicist and popular author Max Tegmark, who is joining the ranks of those who believe they've figured out how to reduce one of science's greatest secrets to numbers. Bits of information to be exact.

Okay, so we now know that the theory is kind of a big deal to notable scientists. But how exactly does IIT attempt to quantify something as ill-defined and seemingly elusive as consciousness?

## IIT in a nutshell

Just like a computer, the brain stores and processes information. But it is how that information is shared throughout the brain network that gives rise to our rich and vivid conscious experience. Let's consider the act of observing a sunset. Thanks to advances in brain imaging, modern neuroscience tells us that there are a number of different and distinct regions active during this event, each of which process information about different features of that event separately. There's a region in the visual cortex (known as "V2") that processes the form and color of the yellow and orange sunrays against the clouds. There are auditory areas in the temporal lobe being fed information about the sound of the wind rushing past you as you stare off into the horizon. That rushing wind against your skin also generates patterns of electrical signals in the somatosensory cortex that create a sense of touch. There are many different things going on in distant places.

Yet somehow we perceive it all as one unified conscious experience.

According to IIT, this unified experience relies on the brain's ability to fuse together (or integrate) all that incoming sensory information as a whole. To measure the degree of integration, Tononi has taken mathematical principles formulated by American engineer Claude Shannon, who developed a scientific theory of information midway through the 20th century to describe data transmission, and applied them to the brain. IIT claims that these information measures allow one to calculate an exact number that represents the degree of integrated information that exists in a brain at any given moment. Tononi chooses to call this metric "Phi" (or Φ), which serves as an index for consciousness. The greater the Phi, the more conscious the system. It need not matter whether it's the nervous system of a child, or a cat, or even a ladybug.

"

"The religion of the future will be a cosmic religion. It should transcend personal God and avoid dogma and theology. Covering both the natural and the spiritual, it should be based on a religious sense arising from the experience of all things natural and spiritual as a meaningful unity."

Albert Einstein

# YOUTUBE
## H O L I S T I C

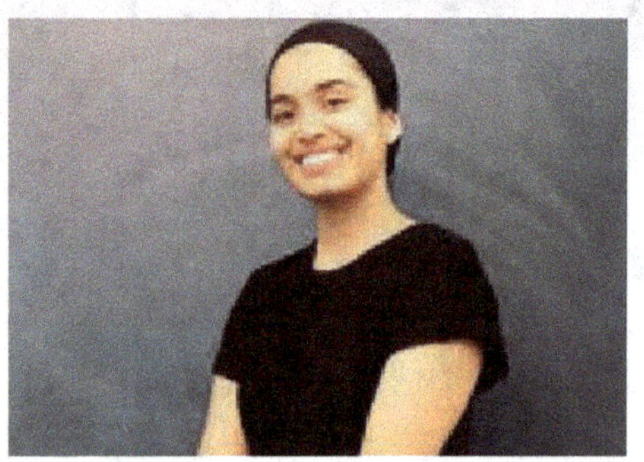

**KAUR HEALTH**

Hey! Meet nutritional coach and personal well being-cheerleader, Jaspreet Kaur. On her channel, she discusses topics like: herbal medicine, diets. health journeys, toxic care products, wholesome recipes and more. Expect to see guests who bare their soul and honestly share their health journey and experiences with dieting/food.

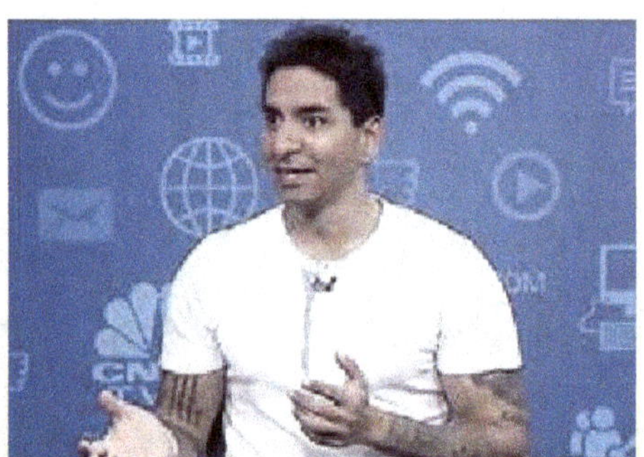

**LUKE COUTINHO**

Luke Coutinho, is a Holistic Nutritionist specialising in the field of Integrative and Lifestyle Medicine. Luke along with his team of qualified Doctors and trained nutritionists design wellness plans with a holistic approach towards prevention, weight and disease management with expertise in cancer care. His programs are personalised and customised according to an individual's lifestyle and revolves around the 4 pillars of good health: Quality Sleep, Balanced Nutrition, Emotional Detox and Adequate Exercise.

His youtube features nutrition, exercise, yoga, meditation, lifestyle medicine and more...

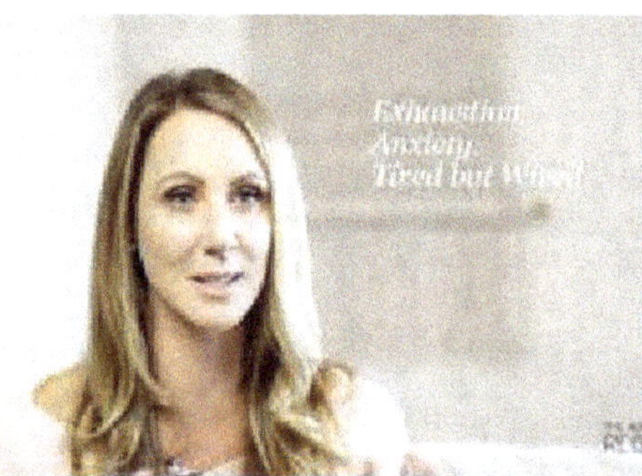

**THE WHOLE JOURNEY.**

The Whole Journey is a clinical and holistic nutritional counseling company. It was created to empower others to take control of their health and vitality using customized whole food nutrition, top quality supplementation and healthy lifestyle guidance. While most dieticians dwell on calories, carbs, fats, proteins, and restrictions, The Whole Journey philosophy is to provide clients with the 'tools' to create a happy, healthy and holistic life in a way that is flexible, fun and free of willpower and denial.

A true holistic approach to life incorporates things that nourish other than food, including honest and open relationships, a meaningful spiritual practice, a career that inspires you, and physical activity that you enjoy. This holistic channel will guide you to make gradual, lifelong changes that enable you to reach your current and future health goals.

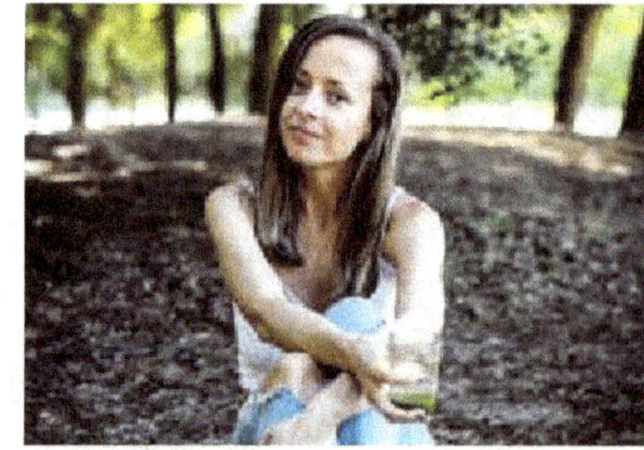

**HOLISTIC WELLNESS PROJECT.**

Marta Tuchowska is a passionate "best-helping", internationally acclaimed health author, self-care coach and wellbeing expert specializing in the alkaline diet lifestyle, mindfulness and mind-body relaxation for holistic wellness.

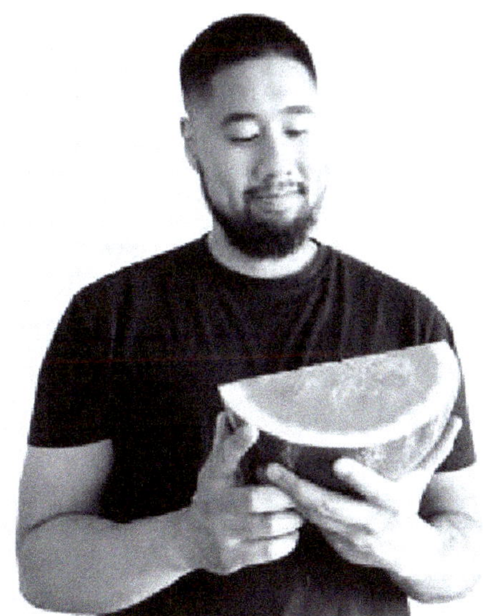

**LIVE IT HOLISTIC NUTRITION**
Marc Capistrano helps people navigate their food journey. His channel is simply a mix of food related content and my everyday life with a focus on exercise and nutrition.

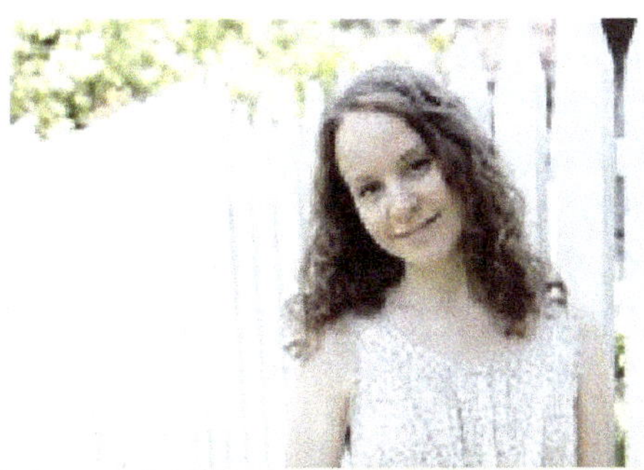

**MEGHAN LIVINGSTONE.**
Meghan is a Certified Holistic Nutritionist, blogger, and a lover of life.

She has a passion for all things healthy, simple and natural. On this channel you will find everything from natural health and wellness tips, minimalism, green beauty & gluten-free, dairy-free recipes.

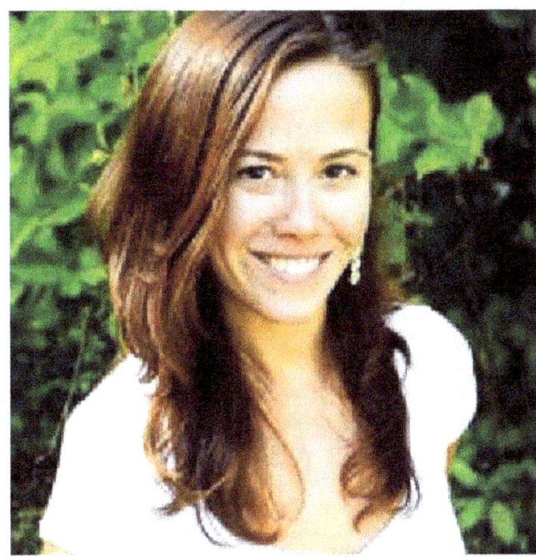

**HEATHER NICHOLDS.**
Heather is a Certified Holistic Nutritionist, an environmentalist, a food lover, a vegan, and an eternal optimist. Her channel features vegan recipes, nutrition advice, motivation, and sometimes eco-tips in my videos, posted on Thursdays.

**HEALTHY LIFE HAPPY LIFE**
This channel is for anyone who wants to live a healthy and positive life with simple, realistic changes that are backed by science. On the channel, you'll see videos on topics such as :

• Eating healthy with easy, practical changes

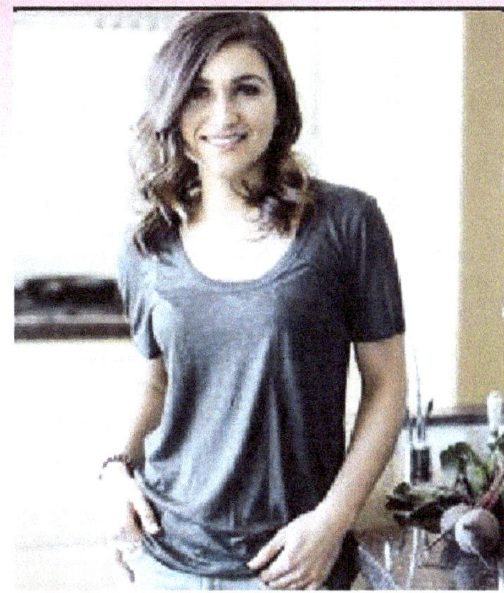

• Living with less (minimalism) + designing a life you love
• Creating a healthier lifestyle with science-backed tips

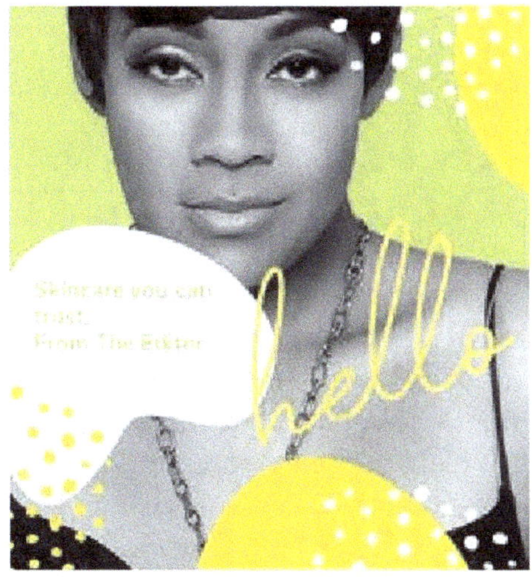


**BEUNIQUE MAGAZINE**
New Holistic lifestyle platform for conscious eating, meditation, spiritual guide, herbal recipes, cooking with herbs, organic and natural anti-aging skincare.

# HOLISTIC BOOKS

### DEEPER THAN BEAUTY

DIY recipes to help you slow down, take care of yourself & your loved ones.

In this book, we will explore the wonders of our gut & skin health, along with the importance & beauty of creating homemade skincare products.

### PLANT BASED FOR BEGINNERS (10 DAY CHALLENGE)

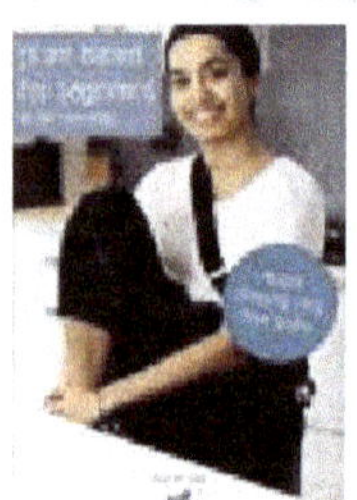

Tranisitioning to a plant-based diet isn't as daunting as you may think! This 10-day transition guide includes recipes, a full 10-day meal plan AND a shopping list to assist you every step of the way. No calorie counting, no restrictions, no fad diets. Just add more nutritious, fibre-rich foods into your diet and see how your body THRIVES!

### THE MAGIC IMMUNITY PILL - LIFESTYLE

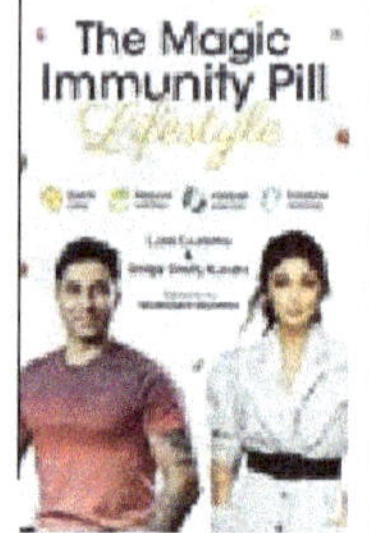


Immunity has become a buzzword now, but it has always been the fundamental of human health and everything revolves around it. Considering how crucial having a strong immunity is at this point, Luke Coutinho and Shilpa Shetty Kundra, put together a book which is a free gift to India and the entire world, with a hope that it will help boost everyone's immune system with basic, inexpensive and simple lifestyle changes

### THE DRY FASTING MIRACLE - FROM DEPRIVE TO THRIVE

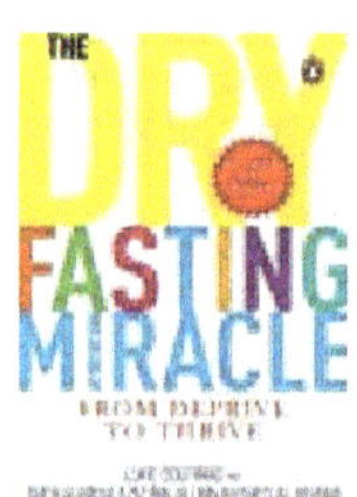


In the olden days, people ate early because there was hardly any light after sunset. Their next meal would only be after sunrise. This practice spread to all religions as a discipline due to its health and spiritual benefits. Today, it is called the dry fasting diet-the most superior form of fasting and cleansing for the body. Replicating it requires abstinence from all food and water for twelve hours or more.

Luke Coutinho and Sheikh Abdulaziz Bin Ali Bin Rashed Al Nuaimi teach us how this diet can stimulate the body, help one find the right balance between the 'elimination phase' and the 'building phase', aid weight loss and help avoid a number of diseases. From beauty to general well-being, discover the miracle of dry fasting and the route to a new you.

### THE MAGIC WEIGHTLOSS PILL

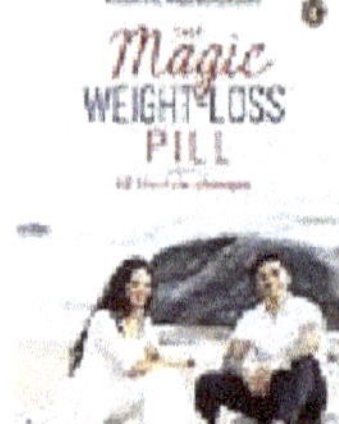


What's the one remedy common to controlling diabetes, hyperthyroidism, kidney and liver stones and excess weight? Lifestyle. Globally renowned holistic lifestyle coach Luke Coutinho and popular Indian actor and Yoga instructor (continuing training with Bharat Thakur, founder of Artistic Yoga) Anushka Shetty are the co-authors of this quintessential book on how to live well and lose weight. This book shows us that nothing parallels the power and impact that simple sustained lifestyle changes can have on a person who's struggling to lose excess weight or suffering from a chronic disease.

### THE GREAT INDIAN DIET

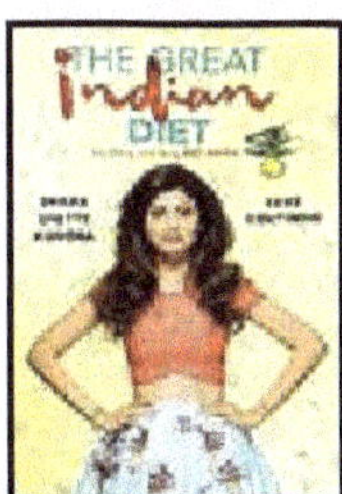


In a world of fads, restrictive diet programs, dangerous exercise plans, unreliable media, and misleading social circles, The Great Indian Diet decodes nutrition and demystifies health and lifestyle from a perspective of simplicity.

The journey of The Great Indian Diet started when Shilpa Shetty and Luke shared a common dream to see people proud of the Indian Diet and to see people use the Indian diet to get healthier.

### EAT SMART, MOVE MORE, SLEEP RIGHT - YOUR PERSONAL HEALTH COACH

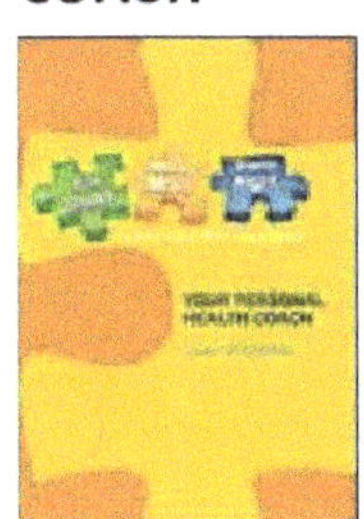

This book is not based on the lifestyles of the rich and famous. It re-acquaints you with the simple, real and inexpensive facts and truths which have always existed - but which have been complicated and twisted by Man. This volume is based on the simple concepts that have transformed hundreds of people's lives in the areas of health, fitness, weight loss, disease and general well-being. Eat Smart. Move More. Sleep Right. contains a 60-day toolkit to achieve the fitness and weight-loss goals you have always desired. Learn how simple it is to get fit, stay healthy and make the lifestyle changes that will last forever. Watch your health and life transform as you learn about these simple facts and the power of the mind.

### ALKALINE GREEN SMOOTHIES

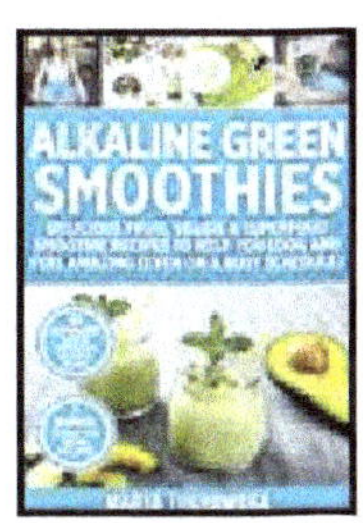


Delicious Fruit, Veggie & Superfood Smoothie Recipes to Help You Look and Feel Amazing (even on a busy schedule) (Alkaline Smoothie Recipes)

"This book makes changing bad eating habits fun!"-
by Moonlily

### ALKALINE JUICING

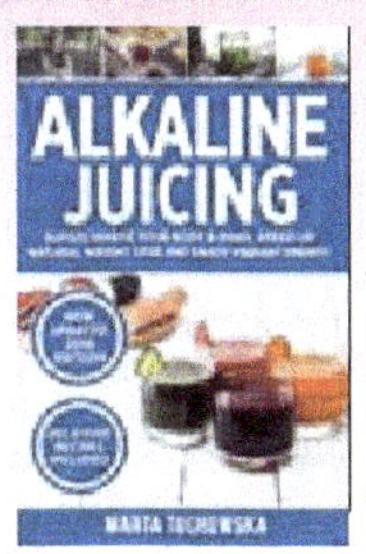


Supercharge Your Body & Mind, Speed Up Natural Weight Loss, and Enjoy Vibrant Energy (Alkaline Drinks, Alkaline Diet for Beginners)

### HOLISTIC SELF-CARE JOURNAL:

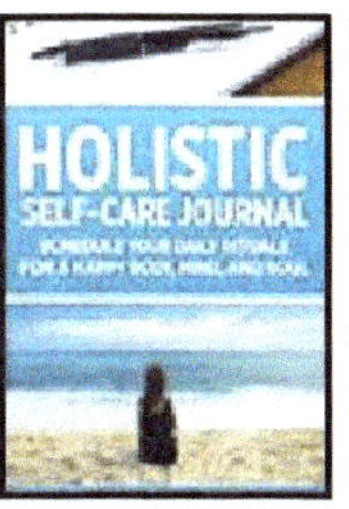


Schedule Your Daily Rituals for a Happy Body, Mind, and Soul. If you want to function at the optimal level and use your wellbeing to enrich all areas of your life, you need to prioritize self-care.
Taking care of your body, mind, and soul will help you feel more energized at work, while at the same time, reducing stress and helping you sleep better.

# SPIRITUAL BOOKS

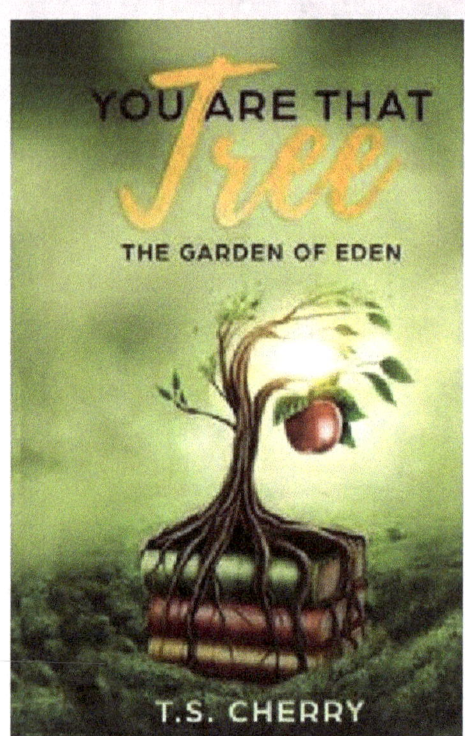


**YOU ARE THAT TREE**
STEP INTO THE NEXT LEVEL OF LIFE!

You are the Tree, an exposé on the two trees in the Garden of Eden, opens up on the power within you, either to be the tree of life - which is the expression of God through flesh - or the tree of good and evil.

The author expounds deeply on the forbidden apple, which is the "way without God; the path of self; the way of disobedience." She explains the consequences of "giving the forbidden apple a bite," which is to make a decision to follow your own path in life, instead of God's.

Learn in this blockbuster messianic book, how you can differentiate between the voice of the snake and that of God, which is the first major struggle of many people. And, how you can put the "snakes" – the wrong voices and influences - out of the garden of your life.

This is your season to step into the next level of life!

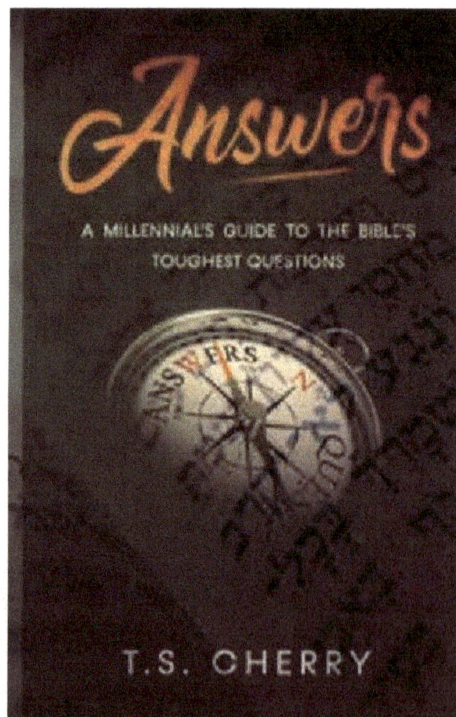


**ANSWERS**
WHY ARE YOU PERSECUTING ME?

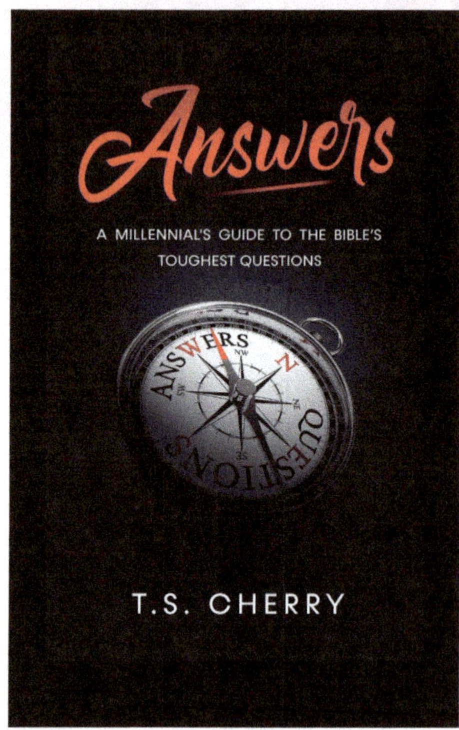


**BREAK YOUR PRESUMPTIONS!**
There are times when you think you're making the right decisions when actually you're making the wrong decisions.

Many times, the people you think are good could be bad and the people you think are bad could be good.

Now, it's time to break your presumptions and encounter better wisdom, better revelation, and better understanding, that will make you a better business person, better husband, better father, and in fact, better everything! Read This Book!

# HOLISTIC PODCAST

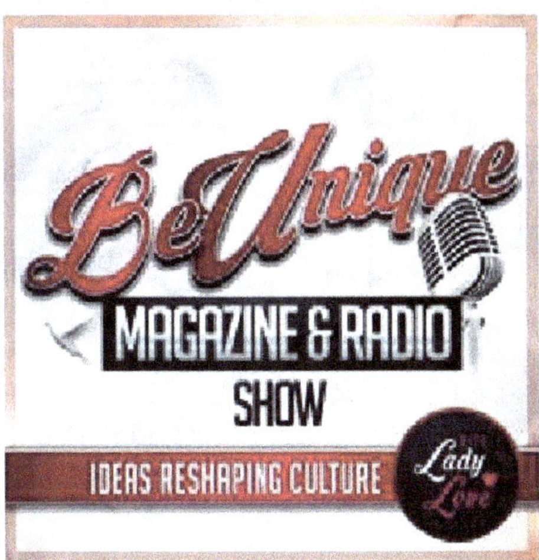


**BeUnique Magazine & Radio Show**
Featuring Holistic News, Holistic segments and more. Take Risks, Find Yourself, Express Yourself! offering a fresh look at the business, and brains, of unique holistic culture.

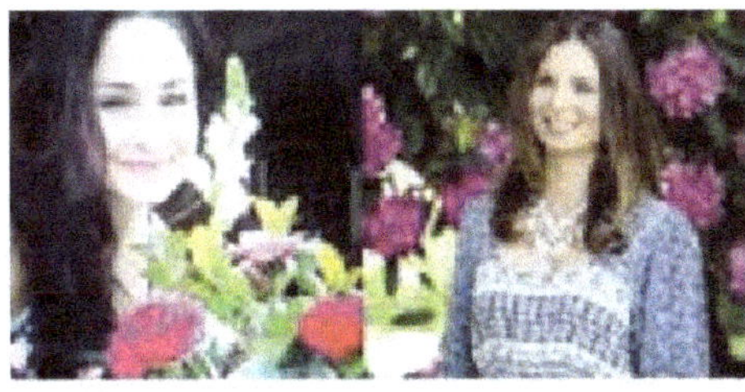

The Holistic Nutritionists
PODCAST

Natalie Bourke & Kate Callaghan

**The Holistic Nutritionists Podcast**
Kate is a Holistic Nutritionist, Personal Trainer and Lifestyle Coach specialising in hormone healing. We also have the most practical tips on holistic health care too. We are always taking podcast questions and topic suggestions.

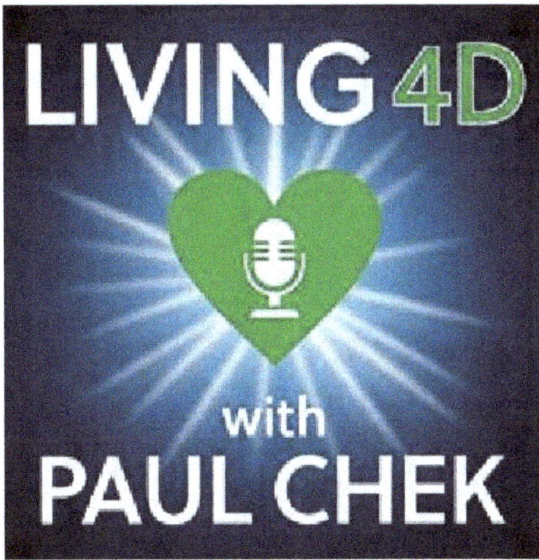


**Living 4D with Paul Chek**
Each week, world-renowned Holistic Health Practitioner Paul Chek and his guests will tackle topics like food, fitness, the environment, science, parenting, the mind, success, religion, love, and sex with a depth and honesty that you won't find anywhere else.

**Holistic Health Masterclass**
Brett is a functional medicine and holistic nutrition practitioner. He is a professional educator and founder of the online education platform, Holistic Health Masterclass. He empower patients and practitioners to live healthier lives and help others to do the same

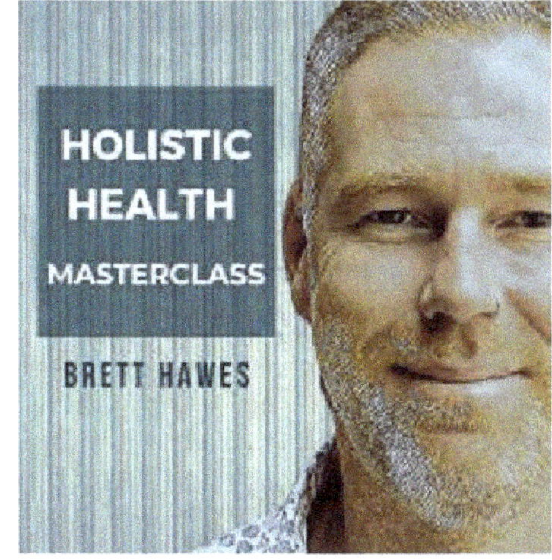


**Holistic Health Masterclass Podcast**
Brett is functional medicine and holistic nutrition practitioner. He is a professional educator and founder of the online education platform, Holistic Health Masterclass. He empowers patients and practitioners to live healthier lives and help others to do the same.

**Holistic Plastic Surgery Show**
In The Holistic Plastic Surgery Show, host and board-certified plastic surgeon Dr. Anthony Youn joins prominent cosmetic surgeons and dermatologists, celebrity health experts, and New York Times best-

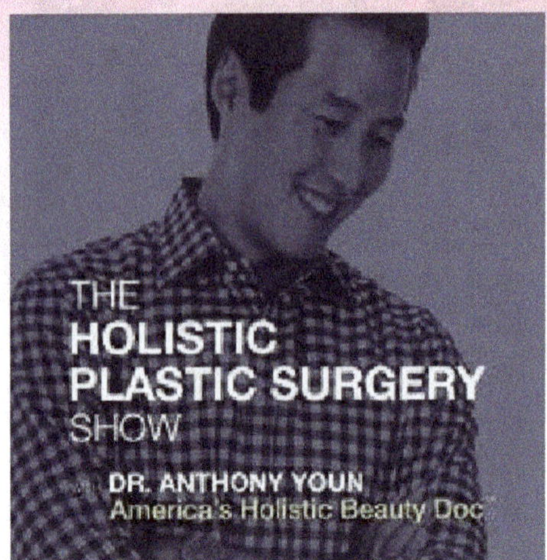


selling authors, to discuss the health topics that matter most to you. They reveal the newest ways to turn back the clock, the latest findings in weight loss and health, and profound insights into living a better life.

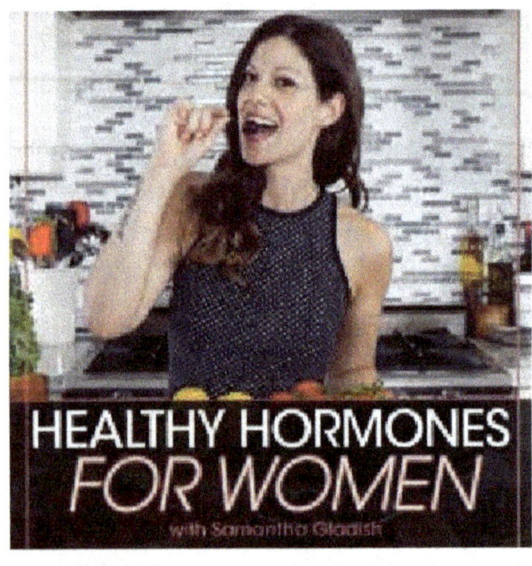


**Healthy Hormones for Women Podcast**
Samantha Gladish from the Holistic Wellness Blog is an Online Nutritionist, Weight Loss Coach and Hormone Fixer-Upper; revealing with you her simple and effective strategies to balancing your hormones, losing weight and creating vibrant health. Discover how you can create more food freedom and more ease, grace and flow in your life to achieve lasting health and vitality.

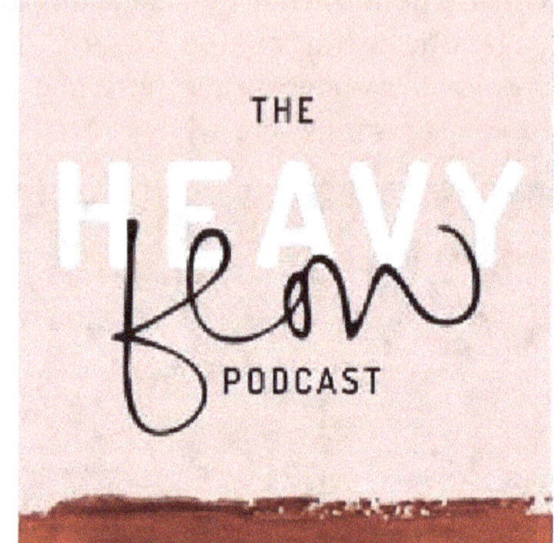


**The Heavy Flow Podcast**
Each week Amanda Laird, Registered Holistic Nutritionist, has casual conversations with guests about the health and wellness topics we're not supposed to talk about: menstruation, fertility, pregnancy, childbirth, menopause, birth control, sexuality, mental health, hormonal health, and reproductive health, through the lenses of feminism and body politics. We are not truly empowered until we all understand the bodies we live in.

**Ronnie Landis**
Ronnie Landis will awaken within you the spark of genius that is your birthright Ronnie Landis is a leading

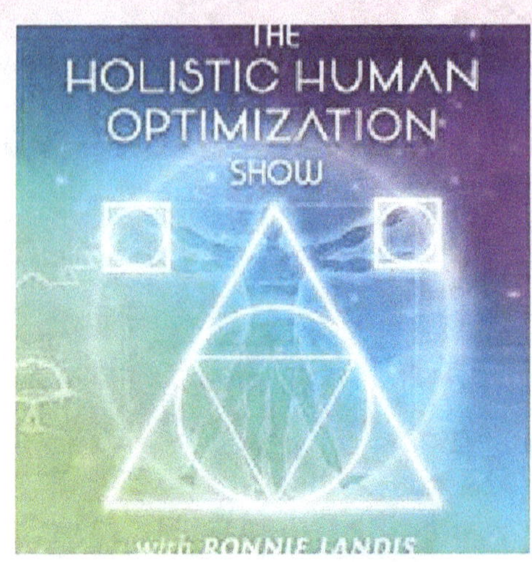


expert in holistic health, natural nutrition, and human potential. He helps people all the way from driven entrepreneurs, athletes, visionary artists.

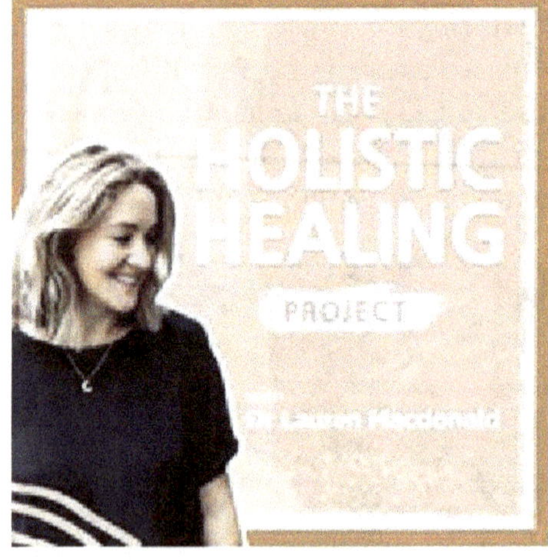


**The Holistic Healing Project**
Each week Lauren talks to experts, thought-leaders and inspiring individuals to explore what HOLISTIC HEALING means to them. Expect raw, honest conversations around health, healing, resilience, mindfulness, personal growth, spirituality and

consciousness. Tune in for tools, guidance and inspiration to guide you towards your healthiest, happiest, most alive and connected self.

We talk about nutrition, natural methods for balancing hormones, understanding your anatomy, menstrual cycles.

powerful actions to understanding keto, developing a ketogenic diet that works for you, overcoming daily keto struggles, boosting body confidence, shedding weight, and more.

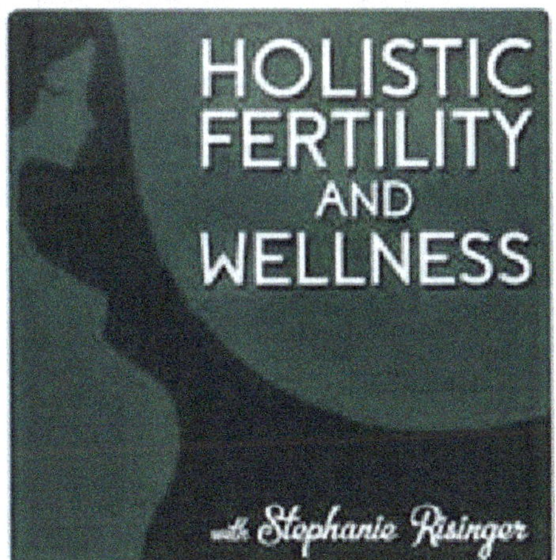


**Holistic Fertility and Wellness**
The Holistic Fertility and Wellness Podcast publishes every other week with episodes running about 30 minutes long. We interview real people like you who have succeeded in their quest for fertility, industry experts & leader, and physicians regarding their thoughts on holistic fertility and best practices for today.

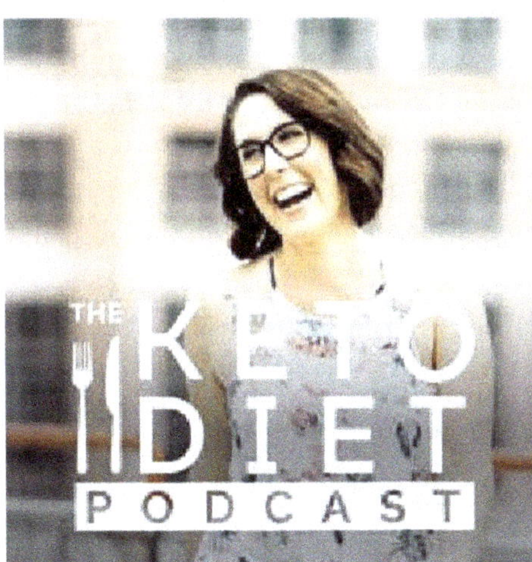


**Healthful Pursuit » The Keto Diet Podcast**
Support your low-carb, high-fat life with The Keto Diet Podcast, a fresh take on ketogenic living with Holistic Nutritionist and keto enthusiast, Leanne Vogel. Interviews with thought leaders, keto veterans, and exclusive content delivering

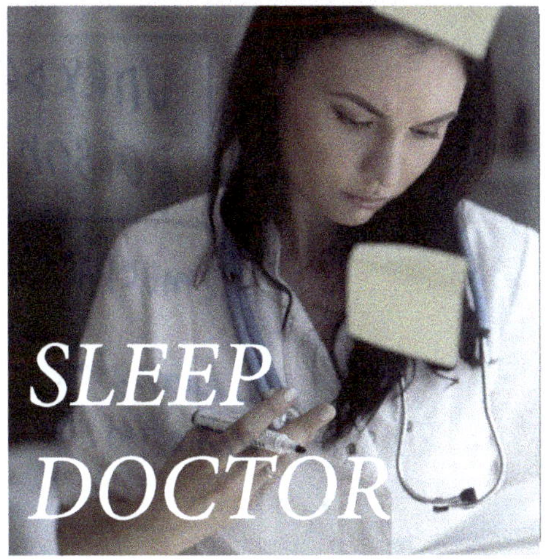


**Holistic Sleep Doc**
Dr. Mike Headlee is The Holistic Sleep Doc who helps people solve their sleep problems without dangerous drugs with a system called the DNA difference. A customized holistic program for people suffering from sleep deprivation and those who want to optimize their sleep.

# AMAZON HOLISTIC

### HOLISTIC HEALTH BASICS

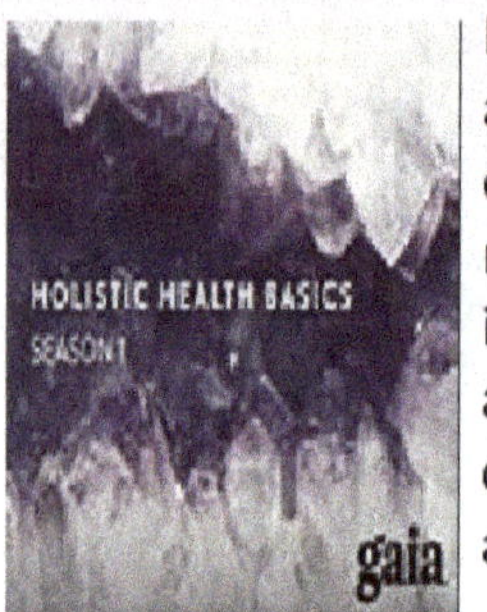


Learn the basics about a variety of holistic modalities, including acupuncture, chinese medicine and Reiki.

### THE DOCTOR FROM INDIA

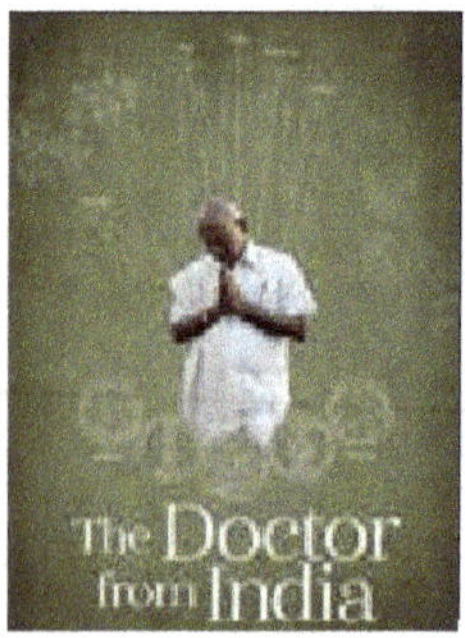


A meditative and immersive portrait of the life and work of Dr. Vasant Lad, the holistic health pioneer who first brought the ancient medical practice of Ayurveda from India to the west in the late 1970s.

### HEALING MATRIX

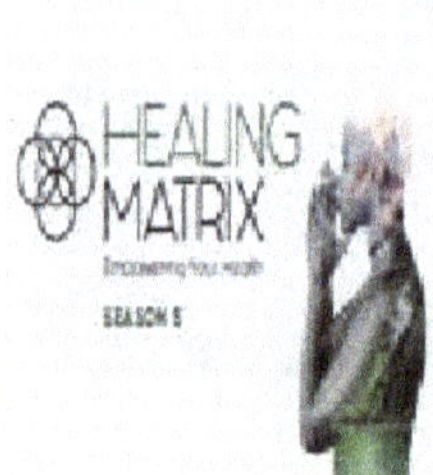


Gain the tools you need to help heal yourself, physically, emotionally and spiritually. Dr. Sue Morter connects you with top researchers and visionaries exploring alternative healing modalities and emerging sciences to bring you information that can help you make better informed choices concerning your health and wellbeing.

### HEALING QUEST

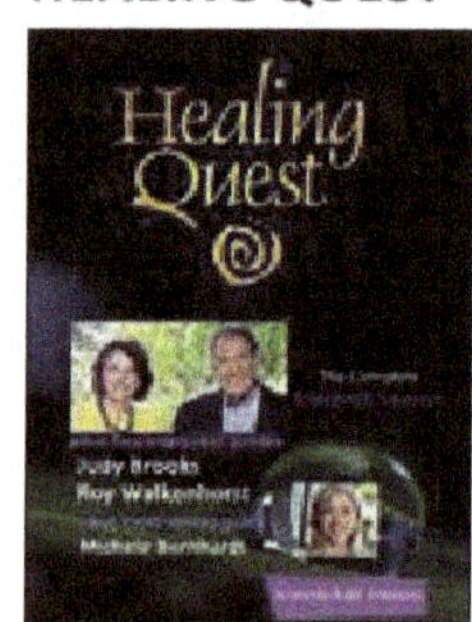


As seen on PBS, HEALING QUEST is based on the booming interest in integrative health and natural approaches to well being. The show subscribes to the philosophy that healing is a lifelong journey toward wholeness, and leading experts explore topics such as alternative medicine, spiritual relaxation, nutrition and diet, physical and mental exercise and socialization.

### INNER WORLDS, OUTER WORLDS

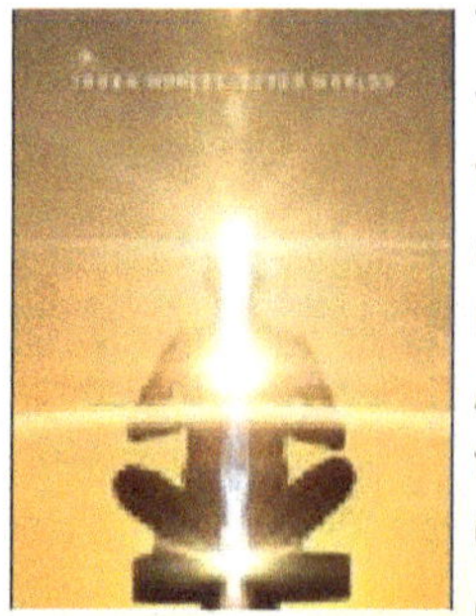

There is one vibratory field that connects all things. It has been called Akasha, Logos, the primordial OM the music of the spheres the Higgs field, dark energy, and a thousand other names. Many of history's monumental thinkers have come to the threshold.

### HOMEOPATHY MYSTERY OF HEALING

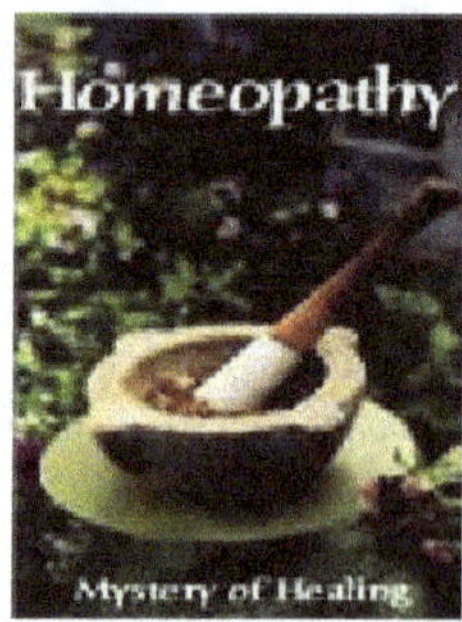


Featuring interviews with experts in the U.S., England, France and Germany, this comprehensive documentary looks at the origins, principles, and modern practice of the alternative and holistic form of medicine known as homeopathy.

### THE LIVING MATRIX

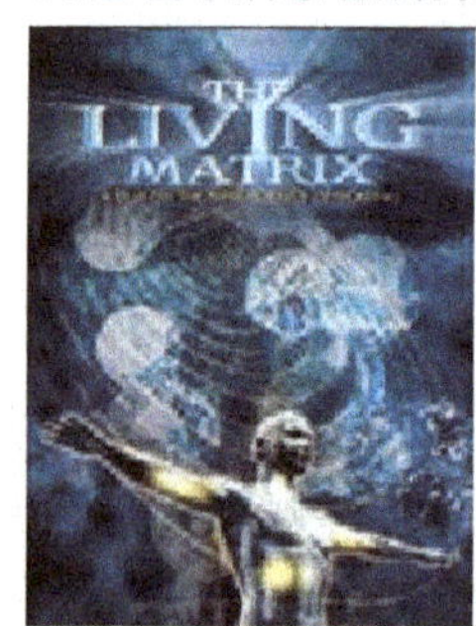


The Living Matrix uncovers new ideas about the intricate web of factors that determine our health. The film features a group of dedicated scientists, psychologists, bioenergetic researchers and holistic practitioners who are finding healing potential in new places.

# HERBAL BLENDS

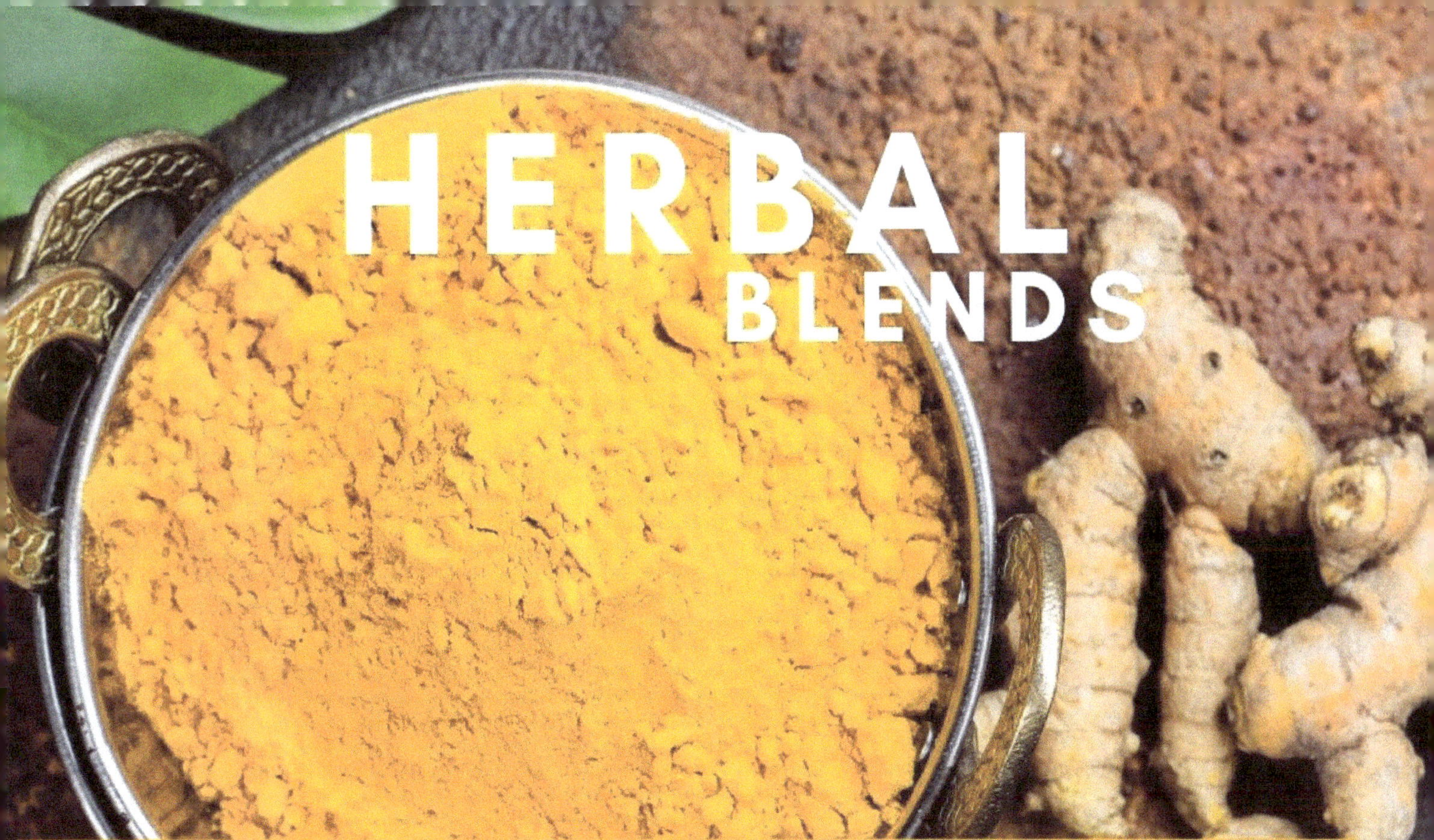

## ABSORPTION

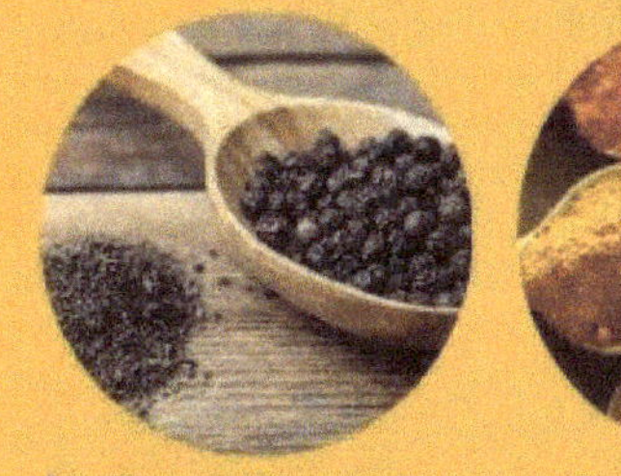

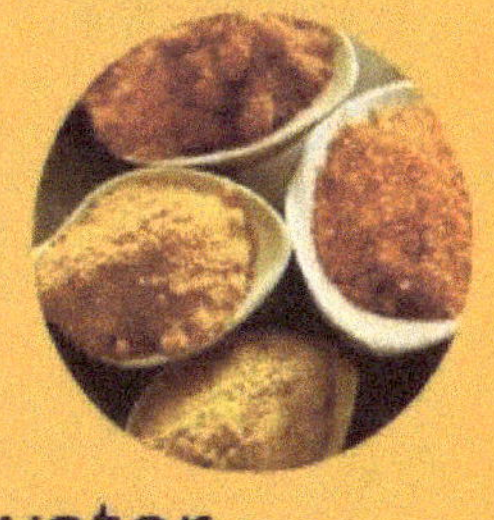

01

PAIRS WELL WITH: Warmed Coconut water, milk based drinks, milk alternatives

**This infused golden blend contains the anti-inflammatory Turmeric and anti-viral Astragalus as a base, with stress reducing adaptogens, for a distinctly potent herbal boost for your gut, skin, and a strong immunizer from the inside out.**

THE APOTHECARY FARMACY

www.ingramcontent.com/pod-product-compliance
Lightning Source LLC
LaVergne TN
LVHW060829170826
845678LV00010B/1935

* 9 7 8 1 9 4 7 0 2 9 1 9 4 *